Natural Weight Management

A Holistic Approach to Sustainable and Healthy Weight Loss

By: Rosemary W. Jones

TABLE OF CONTENTS

Have you noticed that you've gained weight seemingly out of nowhere and without apparent cause? You don't feel as like you've been eating more than usual, and certainly not enough to warrant showing up.

dramatically on the scale.

Almost everyone has gone through this at least once in their life. It surprises us and puts us in a mild state of shock because it doesn't feel like we did anything to earn this extra weight.

I'm not an outlier. I, like millions of others, have gone through the ups and downs of losing and gaining a lot of weight (50 pounds to be exact). There doesn't appear to be any area of health in which there is more time, effort, and money devoted than the subject of weight loss because it is such a pervasive issue.

Thus even when those of us attempting to lose weight cut back on our caloric consumption and increase our exercise, many of us still struggle to lose weight permanently. The typical scenario is to lose weight at first then quickly gain it again. In fact, patients recover all of the weight they lost in around 90% of cases, and frequently end up heavier than when they began!

This book is all about preventing this weight loss roller coaster and assisting you in discovering a method to appreciate weight-loss foods that can help you get and stay small and healthy. A starvation-style diet or one that is nutritionally unbalanced and deprives the body of essential nutrients is something that very few people can maintain. It is becoming more widely accepted that lifestyle changes, such as consuming the World's Healthiest Foods, rather than dieting, are the key to long-term weight loss.

Scientific research is still showing that among every lifestyle

No one component, however, is more crucial to our health than the food we consume. Healthy eating can be easily disregarded as a solution to address our problem of being overweight because the idea of doing so is so unbelievably simple.

The World's Healthiest Foods, for example, are nutrient-rich, health-promoting, and enjoyable foods, and boosting consumption of these foods may be one of the most effective methods to improve wellbeing and achieve healthy weight loss.

Increasing our intake of nutrient-rich foods, such as the World's Healthiest Foods, and reducing our intake of nutrient-poor foods work together to improve our health and promote healthy weight loss. In my book, Healthy Weight Loss - Without Dieting, I emphasize this. I've included a Healthy Weight Loss Eating Plan that takes the guesswork out of preparing 4 weeks' worth of meals that will set you on your way to your weight loss and wellness-fulfilling goals in addition to explaining why nutrient-rich World's Healthiest Food can help you lose weight and improve your health.

You could initially feel starved when you first begin the Plan since you are unable to eat your favorite processed, nutrient-poor meals. However, after two weeks of eating more nutrient-rich foods, you'll notice that your "craving" for these foods will lessen because they'll start to taste too sweet, salty, and fatty. Instead, you'll start to appreciate the more delicate flavors of fresh, whole foods that are high in nutrients, such as the crispiness of fresh salads, the subtle sweetness of blueberries, the robust flavors of high-energy vegetables, and the creamy richness of almonds.

Our key to change may lie in raising public knowledge of the world's healthiest foods. We can begin to view processed, refined meals in a different light as we become more aware of the ingredients they contain. As we perceive them for what they truly are—foods connected to our Healthy Weight Loss — Without Dieting—we will be less drawn to their image of convenience, excitement, and stimulation.

obesity epidemics, immune system impairment, elevated blood sugar levels, increased risk of heart disease, and epidemic levels of obesity all contribute to our propensity for diabetes. To fight your craving for nutrient-poor meals, try eating some of the World's Healthiest Foods.

We can choose from a wide variety of nutrient-dense foods, and gyms and playgrounds can keep us busy and help us burn off those additional calories. When I switched from eating improperly prepared nutrient-poor meals to nutrient-rich World's Healthiest Foods, my health improved, I lost 50 pounds without dieting, and I have kept it off for more than ten years. You too can!

SECTION 1

The foundation of healthy weight loss is nutrient richness.

CHAPTER ONE

The foundation of healthy weight loss is nutrient richness

Nutrient-richness is a measure of the amount of nutrients a food can provide in exchange for the number of calories it contains.

Because we only have a limited number of calories that we can consume if we want to lose or maintain our weight while also taking in a sufficient range and amount of nutrients to maintain our health, it is critical that we get as many nutrients as possible in comparison to the number of calories we consume. Fortunately, focusing on the nutrient-dense World's Healthiest Foods makes this simple.

The most recent scientific research clearly shows that eating nutrient-rich foods is essential for successful weight loss. In large, nationwide studies involving both healthy-weight and overweight participants, inadequate vitamin and mineral intake has consistently been linked to higher body weights. Eating few fresh vegetables and fruits not only results in inadequate nutrition, but it has also been linked to weight problems. Increased consumption of nutrient-rich vegetables has also been linked to better weight loss success in studies of overweight children attempting to lose weight.

Diets high in salads, vegetables, and fruits and low in processed and refined foods are associated with healthy weight because they contain phytonutrients, which are beneficial compounds found exclusively in fruits and vegetables that have the power to keep us healthy and help the body maintain an optimal, healthy weight. Salads, vegetables, and fruits are also high in antioxidants, which we need to lose weight. According to studies, overweight people have higher levels of oxidative stress due to an excess of free radicals and a lack of antioxidants.

What is it about nutrient-dense foods that promotes weight loss?

Several factors are at work. Nutrient-rich World's Healthiest Foods provide our bodies with exceptional nutrient support, allowing our bodies to carry out their metabolic activities optimally. Metabolic activities, such as the burning of unwanted fat (a process known as beta-oxidation), are best supported by a nutrient-dense diet.

Because we only have a limited number of calories to consume if we want to lose or maintain our weight while also taking in a sufficient range and amount of nutrients to maintain our health, it is critical that we get as many nutrients as possible in comparison to the number of calories we consume.

Fortunately, focusing on the nutrient-dense World's Healthiest Foods makes this simple.

The Nutrients We Require Every Day

Every day, we require hundreds of nutrients to maintain our health, and these nutrients must be obtained from the food we consume.

The chart below will give you an idea of the variety of nutrients we need to get each day from our food if we want to maintain a healthy weight and be in good health. Please keep in mind that this chart is not exhaustive; it does not show you all of the nutrients you require.

For example, phytonutrients—plant nutrients such as carotenoids (beta carotene, lutein, zeaxanthan) and flavonoids (anthocyanins, catechins, quercetin)—are now known to be essential to health, but researchers estimate that at least 40,000 phyonutrients may eventually be catalogued.

Even though they have not yet been named or identified in the laboratory, these phytonutrients are still present— in nutrient-rich foods such as the World's Healthiest Foods. In fact, that is the only place you can get them right now! They can't be obtained from dietary supplements, for example, because they haven't yet been isolated from the whole, natural foods that contain them. They are also not found in highly processed "fast" foods.

Fresh fruits and vegetables, as well as salads, are among the most nutrient-dense foods.

It is obvious that nutrient-richness is essential for maintaining health and losing weight in a healthy manner. And what are some of the most nutrient-dense foods that people can easily incorporate into their Healthiest Way of Eating to improve their health? Fruits, salads, and vegetables that are fresh.

However, which foods do most of us not consume enough of? Fruits, salads, and vegetables that are fresh.

In fact, by failing to eat enough fresh fruits, salads, and vegetables, 80% of Americans jeopardize their ability to maintain a healthy weight and jeopardize their health. This is very concerning to me. It's simple: the more fruits, salads, and vegetables you eat, the easier it will be to get the nutrients you need for optimal health at a "caloric cost" that is so low that you will easily lose excess weight. I believe that one of the major causes of the obesity epidemic in this country is Americans' apparent aversion to whole fruits, salads, and vegetables (and, in the Healthy Healthy Weight Loss — Without Dieting Weight Loss Eating Plan, I will show you how to make these foods taste good so that you will truly enjoy them).

My approach to healthy weight loss focuses on fresh fruits, salads, and vegetables—the world's lowest calorie food group. We profile over two dozen low-calorie vegetables and over twenty fruits on the WHFoods.org website and in The World's Healthiest Foods book. With simple recipes and menus based on low-calorie, deliciously prepared fresh fruits, salads, and vegetables, I will assist you in meeting the 5-9 recommended servings per day. These foods, according to weight loss research, are your best option for increasing food volume and enjoying tasty, satisfying meals while keeping your overall calories low.

CHAPTER TWO

Why the World's Healthiest Nutrient-Rich Foods are the Key to Good Health and Weight Loss

Nutrients are the ingredients for health in the body

In this chapter, I'll go over why the nutrients found in the World's Healthiest Foods are so important for your health. You'll see how they offer so many great advantages and are thus the key to healthy weight loss and optimal health.

Although most people are familiar with the concept of nutrition and nutrients, many people do not fully understand what nutrients do and how they work, including how they contribute to weight loss. I'd like to explain what nutrients do by using the simple example of calcium.

You've probably heard that calcium is essential for bone health. You may have also heard that osteoporosis, a bone disease that affects 20 million adults in the United States, can be "prevented by calcium."

I wish things were that easy! However, this is not the case. Even though calcium is essential for bone health, it is simply not true that calcium can prevent osteoporosis on its own.

To begin with, bones require many more nutrients to maintain their structure and density. For example, magnesium, manganese, zinc, vitamin D, vitamin C, vitamin K, boron, silicon, potassium, and a variety of other nutrients are required for good bone health. Simply focusing on calcium will not get you to your goal of good bone health. You require a much broader range of nutrients, which can only be obtained from nutrient-rich foods such as the World's Healthiest Foods.

Most people are used to thinking about nutrients in a "this cures that" type of way. The overly simplified positioning of dietary supplements in the marketplace can sometimes encourage this way of thinking. On product labels, manufacturers frequently include health claims that present relatively simple cause-and-effect relationships between nutrients and health. For example, a supplement manufacturer may claim that calcium promotes bone strength, fiber promotes bowel regularity, or vitamin E promotes heart health.

While all of these links between nutrients and health are scientifically valid, consumers may come to believe that vitamin E is all they need for a healthy heart, or that calcium is all they need for strong bones. The truth is that no single nutrient is a magic bullet that can prevent a disease or protect an entire body system, such as blood vessels or bones.

It's not as if a nutrient can wave a magic wand and fix a health problem. The role that nutrients play in all of the body's underlying structures and metabolic activities is why they are linked to the prevention of future health problems and the improvement of existing ones. They are the resources that our bodies require in order to create and maintain healthy cells. They are the substances that help our metabolism run and allow our bodies to go about their daily physiologic activities. Our bodies cannot function without them: for example, our cells cannot communicate, our muscles cannot contract, and oxygen cannot be carried in our blood. These three activities are joined by literally thousands of other activities that take place every second at a metabolic level that is invisible to us but vital to our health.

Nutrients are thus the ingredients in the body's recipe for Nutrient-Rich Food. The Healthiest Foods in the World Supporting its underlying structure and function, which serve as the foundation for our physical health, is critical to healthy weight loss.

Take any single nutrient and examine everything it does in the body to get a sense of this massive underlying health foundation. Take magnesium as an example.

Magnesium is an enzymatic cofactor in over 300 different reactions.

Many steps in the energy production cycle, as well as the synthesis of our DNA, are included. Magnesium is also an important component of bone structure and is involved in cell-to-cell communication, particularly between nerve and muscle cells.

Our bodies wouldn't be able to function properly if we didn't have enough magnesium, which can first cause fatigue and then potentially progress to a variety of different signs, symptoms, and health conditions when things aren't working properly. As you can see, it's more complicated than simply claiming that magnesium promotes heart health or bone health, two claims that are frequently associated with this mineral. Magnesium, like all other nutrients, is required in hundreds of different ways to support our underlying metabolic processes, which serve as the true foundation for our overall physical health.

You might think that taking a more comprehensive and holistic approach to health and nutrition would make nutrition more difficult.

But it's the exact opposite! The true role of nutrients in your health actually simplifies things.

This is because the World's Healthiest Foods are also comprehensive and holistic! When you look at the World's Healthiest Foods as a whole, you'll notice that their nutrients help with every aspect of our metabolic and cellular needs. They not only maintain this massive underlying biochemical structure that supports all of our health, but they do so in the most natural way possible by combining nutrients in their most natural patterns. No supplement will ever achieve this incredible level of nutrient synergy! All you have to do is focus on enjoying the World's Healthiest Foods because their nutrient-richness and natural synergy of nutrients will do the rest of the work for you.

Why Is It Difficult to Maintain a Healthy Weight When You Don't Eat Enough Nutrient-Rich Food? The Healthiest Foods in the World

The modern American diet is frequently criticized as being prone to excess. Too many calories, too many fats, too many sweets, too much fried food, too much salt, too much meat! Many health experts see obesity in this light: as a problem caused by excess and overconsumption.

However, the opposite side of the equation in terms of health and maintaining a healthy weight—underconsumption and nutrient deficiency—is also true. The American diet is full of deficiencies and malnutrition.

What happens when our nutrient intake is this low? If it's only for a few days, there's usually nothing to worry about. When we are healthy, our bodies have nutrient reserves from which to draw to meet our nutritional requirements.

However, if we are nutrient deficient week after week, month after month, this can set us on the path to chronic disease and unhealthy weight gain. Developing a serious illness as a result of nutrient deficiency is a slow and gradual process.

We used to think of nutrient deficiency conditions as involving the complete absence of a single nutrient and the emergence of unusual symptoms fairly quickly. A good example is the disease scurvy, which is caused by a lack of vitamin C.

This condition, which is easily visible in the form of gum damage, was first observed in sailors on long voyages without the benefit of fruits and vegetables on board.

In this case, there is a fairly new and direct link between a single nutrient deficiency (vitamin C) and a very specific set of symptoms (damage to the gums).

Today's nutrient deficiency diseases do not follow the scurvy pattern. Today, not a single nutrient intake level has fallen below the recommended level. It is more like a dozen nutrients because we consume all of them in far insufficient amounts. We may not see any visible signs of disease related to these nutrient deficiencies over a period of several years.

Instead, we may simply feel tired more frequently than we should. Or that we don't sleep as well as we should, or that we don't feel well rested when we wake up. Or that we are tired and unable to concentrate.

Our chronic nutrient deficiency is undoubtedly leading us to more serious health problems, even if we have yet to see visible evidence of these problems.

Long-term nutrient deficiency alters the way our bodies function beneath the surface, at the cellular level. Almost all bodily functions necessitate specific nutrient combinations. Without vitamin E, we cannot maintain the integrity of our cell membranes. Without copper, zinc, and selenium, we cannot protect the structures inside the cell from oxygen-related damage. Manganese is required for energy production in our cells' mitochondria. Without a specific combination of B-complex vitamins, our muscles cannot use carbohydrates as fuel. All of these processes are disrupted by chronic nutrient deficiency.

They do not stop completely, but rather continue to operate in a suboptimal manner. What begins as suboptimal progresses to fully problematic over time.

Obesity and virtually all chronic diseases have nutrient deficiency as a well-studied contributing factor. (In addition, many commonly consumed, processed foods that can increase our risk of chronic disease can also increase our risk of obesity.) These nutrient deficiencies are clearly associated with cardiovascular disease and include vitamins B6, B12, and folate. The role of nutrient deficiency in diabetes is not as clear as it is in cardiovascular disease, but biotin, magnesium, vitamin E, coenzyme Q, and lipoic acid have all been implicated in animal studies as nutrients that may contribute to disease risk when chronically deficient in the body. When it comes to nutrient deficiency and chronic disease, a long list of anti-inflammatory nutrients, including flavonoids and carotenoids found in most fresh fruits and vegetables, is becoming a particular area of focus. Because so many chronic diseases and obesity appear to have an inflammatory component, a lack of these anti-inflammatory nutrients may be especially important.

As you can see, the link between nutrient deficiency and chronic disease is not simple, straightforward, or obvious. But the take-home message here is clear: if we want to reduce our risk of chronic disease and obesity, we must do everything we can to avoid nutrient deficiency in our meal plans.

That's where the list of the World's Healthiest Foods comes in. They supply you with all of the nutrients you require for good health. And with the Healthy Weight Loss Eating Plan, you'll see how simple it is to eat a variety of these foods to make delicious meals while getting all of the nutrients you need for health and avoiding nutrient deficiency or malnutrition.

We'll go over nutrients and health in greater detail in the following chapter. We'll look at why they're so important for healthy weight loss and overall health.

SECTION 2

Why Are the World's Healthiest Nutrient-Rich Foods Important for Healthy Weight Loss

CHAPTER THREE

Why Is It Important to Eat the World's Healthiest Nutrient-Rich Foods for Healthy Weight Loss?

Adverse food reactions (also known as "food allergies") can cause a variety of symptoms and can be the root cause of health problems. These adverse food reactions are more common than you might think, and they can be surprisingly difficult to identify as contributing factors to health problems. Food allergies that begin in childhood and continue throughout life are examples of adverse food reactions. They can also include more transient reactions to food that occur when you are particularly tired and your physical health is compromised. In either case, you will not always have an obvious symptom that says, "Aha! My body is reacting negatively to something I ate." In the case of adverse food reactions, you are much more likely to feel bad in some way (e.g., fatigued, irritable, depressed, foggy headed, lethargic) due to a variety of causes. All of the symptoms listed above, for example, could be caused by a lack of sleep, chronic stress, or a variety of other psychological factors.

When we have an adverse food reaction, we may be reacting to multiple food components. It's possible that some unusual food proteins are causing our problems. It's also possible that we don't have enough enzymes to digest sugars in our diet.

We may also be sensitive to food additives and preservatives, as well as pesticides and other food contaminants.

Regardless of the food component causing an adverse reaction, you will almost always feel better if you can eliminate the food from your meal plan (or at the very least significantly reduce your consumption of the food). As you will see later in this chapter, this process of avoiding potentially problematic foods is commonly referred to as a "elimination diet." Later in this chapter, I'll go over the specifics of a modified elimination diet that you can incorporate into your own meal planning as you strive for weight loss and better health.

Adverse food reactions are caused by a mismatch between a person and a food. We might not be built to eat anything and everything! You may have a more difficult time losing weight if you and your food are mismatched. Recent reviews of popular weight loss diets clearly show that unusual diets are unsupportive of weight loss when compared to balanced, metabolically matched diets. Although adverse food reactions have not been specifically studied in this regard, they have been established as real-life responses to food that can upset many different metabolic balances in a person's body, as well as compromise function in several different body systems, including the digestive system, immune system, nervous system, endocrine system, and inflammatory system. Your path to healthy and optimal weight loss will be jeopardized if these body systems are not functioning properly.

Dairy and wheat are two important examples of adverse food reactions that are not specifically linked to weight management issues but are relatively high on most research lists of foods most likely to cause adverse reactions. Here's a closer look at each of those foods and the risks associated with them.

In the case of dairy, up to 15% of all infants in the United States exhibit unwanted reactions to cow's milk, including common symptoms that can be attributed to a variety of other factors other than food. Irritability, fussiness, upset stomach, and bowel problems such as excessive gas, bloating, or diarrhea are among the symptoms. However, when tested for food allergies, as few as 5% of all infants test positive for cow's milk allergy. Some studies estimate that the prevalence of dairy allergy in adults is similar to that of children, while others estimate that it is slightly lower. (As with all food allergies, we don't have very accurate data to estimate how many people are actually affected.)

In the case of dairy, the adverse reaction is sometimes caused by milk sugar (lactose). Lactase, an enzyme that breaks down milk sugar and allows it to be digested properly, is not present in all people.

Unfortunately, milk sugar (lactose) is frequently added to non-dairy foods for flavor in the processed food industry, and the only way to avoid it is to read the ingredient list on the package. Lactose can be found in foods such as sliced deli meats, powdered coffee creamers, and ready-to-eat baked goods. Many people are allergic to caseins, which are special proteins found in cow's milk. Unfortunately, in the world of processed foods, these proteins can be found in a wide variety of foods in forms such as calcium caseinate or sodium caseinate. Casein can be found in foods such as hot dogs, deli meats, nutrition bars, and protein powder drinks. Individuals who have adverse reactions to dairy frequently believe that their entire dietary balance has been compromised. The consequences of consuming dairy can detract from the satisfaction of eating or cause confusion about the diet's trustworthiness.

Weight management challenges often become more difficult in these circumstances.

There is even less conclusive research on adverse food reactions in the case of wheat than there is for dairy. However, scientists are continuing to look into the relationship between specific wheat proteins, such as gliadin proteins and lectins (particularly WGA, or wheat germ agglutinin), and their ability to cause adverse reactions. Wheat components, like lactose and casein in dairy, find their way into many types of processed foods, and it is possible to have an adverse reaction to wheat even if you do not eat foods like wheat bread and wheat pasta that are clearly identifiable as wheat containing foods. Soy sauce, teriyaki sauce, and seasoning mixes are examples of processed foods that may contain wheat components; common processed food ingredients such as malt (including barley malt and malt extract) may also contain wheat components. Adverse reactions to wheat, like those to dairy, can make people feel as if their entire dietary balance has been thrown off, making weight management more difficult.

Dietary Elimination

I've seen how adverse food reactions can make losing weight difficult. As a result, if you find that after three weeks of focusing your diet on enjoying the World's Healthiest Foods, you haven't lost any weight, you may want to investigate whether adverse food reactions are to blame.

In this case, I would recommend a modified elimination diet. Keeping a journal is one of the best tools for this. Write down all of the foods you eat at each meal, and then when you reintroduce eliminated foods, note whether or not you have an adverse reaction to them.

I understand that you will need the assistance of a licensed healthcare practitioner to diagnose or treat a food allergy, as well as the assistance of a healthcare practitioner to embark on a full-fledged, nutritionally restrictive or nutritionally complicated elimination diet. (I should also mention that in the case of some full-fledged elimination diets, medical monitoring is essential for safety.) In this case, however, I am not referring to a full-fledged elimination diet. I'm only mentioning some practical steps you can take to experiment with avoiding foods that are commonly linked to adverse food reactions.

The foods listed below are less likely to be associated with these types of problematic reactions.

- Cabbage
- Carrots
- Celery
- Salad greens
- Garlic
- Green beans
- Green peas
- Kale
- Extra virgin olive oil
- Onions
- Lettuce
- Squash in the summer (zucchini)

- Yummy sweet potatoes
- Chard (Swiss chard)
- Apples
- Grapes
- Lemons
- Pears
- Rice (brown)
- Black beans
- Garbonzo beans
- Lentils
- Cauliflower seeds
- toasted sesame seeds
- Seeds of sunflower
- Cod
- Lamb
- Salmon

You must determine how comfortable you are with limiting your food intake to the above list. If you are concerned about staying well-nourished on the foods listed above, you should consult with a healthcare practitioner before making these dietary changes on your own.

You won't notice many changes in your health or well-being unless you stick with these food modifications for at least one week, so you should feel comfortable sticking to this restricted meal plan for that long. After one week, you should begin re-introducing old foods into your meal plan. I recommend that you only introduce one food at a time and wait at least two days before reintroducing another. When beginning this food re-introduction process, I would also recommend starting with asparagus, avocados, beets, broccoli, Brussels sprouts, cauliflower, cucumbers, blueberries, watermelon, flaxseeds, and quinoa because they are not as commonly associated with adverse food reactions as some of the other foods you may have eliminated from your meal plan.

Following that, you should continue reintroducing other foods into your meal plan one at a time, waiting at least two days before adding the next food. Try to notice any adverse reactions as you reintroduce the foods that you avoided during your week on the modified elimination diet. Pay close attention to any issues that prompted you to try food elimination in the first place. If these issues reoccur, it may indicate that the newly reintroduced food is not well-suited to your body's metabolism and should be avoided in future meal planning.

If you suspect any adverse reactions while using this modified elimination method, you should consult with a nutritionist or other healthcare provider who has extensive experience with food allergies.

CHAPTER FOUR

The World's Healthiest Foods Help Energy Production

We all want more energy—usually all the time, but especially when it comes to losing weight. It's common to feel drained of energy when we change our eating habits or reduce our overall caloric intake. It is now more important than ever for our food to provide us with that extra energy boost.

One reason nutrient-rich World's Healthiest Foods are so beneficial is that they help you feel energized while losing weight.

And here's how it works: the World's Healthiest Foods can help you energize by providing your body with adequate amounts of nutrients required by the body's energy production systems.

It's not just that they provide you with enough macronutrients (carbohydrates, protein, and fat) to get your metabolism going. They also contain micronutrients (vitamins and minerals) that aid in the release of energy and its recapture for later use when and where it is most needed.

Your cells are responsible for capturing energy from the food you eat.

The mitochondria, which are very small microstructures inside our cells, are some of the most important energy production sites. The energy production process that occurs in our mitochondria is a complex one. It requires many vital health-promoting nutrients, such as vitamins B1, B2, B3, B5, and B6, lipoic acid, coenzyme Q, and iron, magnesium, and sulfur, to function properly. Consider how much energy you'll have if you eat nutrient-poor refined foods instead of nutrient-rich whole foods like fresh fruits, salads, and vegetables. These and other World's Healthiest Foods will undoubtedly supply your energy systems with the health-promoting nutrients they require to fuel your vitality.

Furthermore, nutrient-dense World's Healthiest Foods, particularly fruits and vegetables, contain phytonutrients that act as powerful antioxidants. These plant-based nutrients have the ability to support healthy energy production, in addition to many other benefits. Because your body generates oxygen radicals while producing energy, which can damage the mitochondrial energy centers as well as many cells and tissues, resulting in reduced and inefficient energy production. However, phytonutrients and other antioxidants (such as vitamin E) found in nutrient-dense World's Healthiest Foods can act as protective sentries for your cells, quenching oxygen radicals and preventing them from causing damage.

CHAPTER FIVE

The World's Healthiest Foods Encourage Optimal Metabolism

Weight loss that is healthy involves the burning of body fat while preserving other tissue (such as muscle mass). While "fat burning" may appear to be a simple process, it is far from it.

In chemistry, "fat burning" refers to the oxidation of fat. Many different enzymes and nutrients are required to break down body fat and convert it to energy. Vitamins B2 (riboflavin), B3 (niacin), and B5 are directly involved in this process (pantothenic acid).

Proteins, as well as sulphur and phosphorus-containing molecules, are also involved. We will not burn body fat optimally if our food does not provide us with an adequate supply of these fat-metabolizing nutrients. That is why, when looking to optimize healthy weight loss, it is critical to focus on nutrient-rich World's Healthiest Foods—for their concentration of these and other nutrients.

There is also preliminary research on the role of specific nutrients in causing "thermogenesis" in brown fat cells. The World's Healthiest Foods, particularly those high in protein and low in refined carbohydrates, as well as those high in fiber, are critical for activating thermogenic heat production in brown adipose (fat) cells. Furthermore, they reduce the storage of dietary fat in ordinary cells; thus, they may be beneficial factors to consider in the process of weight loss or any aspect of weight management.

I'd like to draw your attention to another area of research involving optimal metabolism and weight loss: contamination of whole, natural foods with pesticides and other toxic substances when these foods are grown and processed in an unhealthy manner. Some preliminary evidence suggests that chlorine-containing pesticides and other compounds (collectively referred to as "organochlorines") can disrupt thermogenesis and make weight loss more difficult. By emphasizing organically grown foods, you can avoid these organochlorine contaminants! You won't have to worry about them interfering with your body's metabolism if you stick to organically grown whole foods as much as possible.

CHAPTER SIX

The World's Healthiest Foods Aid Digestive Health

The World's Healthiest Foods supply our digestive system with the nutrients it requires to function optimally. This is critical not only for overall health but also for successful weight loss.

To achieve healthy weight loss, we must maintain metabolic energy supplies to our brain, muscles, and other organ systems. This "metabolic maintenance" is only possible when the digestive tract is functioning properly. Your digestive tract is the starting point for everything.

When you chew your food, you start the digestive process. It is critical to chew thoroughly in order to break down the food into small enough pieces for proper digestion. I believe that the more you chew, the more weight you will be able to lose. Nutrients will not be available for absorption into your body unless you can effectively break down your food. And if you can't absorb the nutrients, they can't help the rest of your body. If you want to lose weight in a healthy way, you must be able to digest food and absorb nutrients properly.

As I will discuss in Chapter 10, maintaining inflammatory balance in the body may be especially important during times of weight loss.

One way to keep this balance is to ensure that your digestive tract is working properly. Because if your digestion is compromised, unwanted molecules (such as toxic residues or allergy-causing substances) can sometimes enter your bloodstream and trigger unwanted inflammatory responses.

While all nutrients are essential for digestive health, the following are a few of the health-promoting nutrients found in the World's Healthiest Foods that have been singled out for their unique contribution.

Dietary fiber
Dietary fiber is at the top of many lists for digestive tract support.

Food cannot pass through you in an optimal manner unless it contains fiber. We should ideally consume at least 10 grams of fiber with each meal and at least 5 grams with each snack, though 20 grams per meal and 10 grams per snack would also be beneficial to the majority of our digestive tracts. Fiber must be obtained from whole, unprocessed foods. World's Healthiest Foods like vegetables, legumes (like beans or lentils), and whole grains are especially important. Fruit skins are also high in fiber. fiber keeps food moving through our intestines at a steady pace that is neither too fast nor too slow.

Glutamine: Although it is less well known in the conventional nutrition world, glutamine is an amino acid that serves as one of the primary fuels for the cells that line our small intestine. It can be synthesized from other amino acids found in food or our bodies, but it can also be found preformed in a variety of World's Healthiest Foods, such as cabbage, beets, beef, chicken, fish, beans, and dairy products.

Fatty Acids with a Short Chain

Short chain fatty acids (or SCFAs), like glutamine, are not well known in the conventional world of nutrition, but these essential nutrients serve as preferred fuels for the cells that line our large intestine. These cells cannot properly process our food if they lack sufficient energy. SCFAs are formed in our small intestine by bacteria that process starches (especially resistant starches) and other carbohydrate-related molecules found in our food. Whole grains like corn, oats, wheat, rye, and brown rice; fruits like apples and citrus fruits and all legumes are high in resistant starch and non-starch carbohydrates that our intestinal bacteria can convert into SCFAs.

Other Nutrients for Digestive Health

The digestion and absorption process is complex, involving dozens of different cell types, dozens of different enzymes, the movement of smooth muscles around our intestines, and the activation of these muscles by our nerves. There isn't a single vitamin or mineral that doesn't play a role in some aspect of digestive health, either directly or indirectly. As a result, foods with the highest concentration of nutrients and the greatest variety of nutrients are best for digestive support. The World's Healthiest Foods perfectly fit this description because they were all chosen for their nutrient-richness. They supply our digestive tract with all of the nutrients it requires while avoiding putting undue strain on the digestive tract.

CHAPTER SEVEN

The World's Healthiest Foods Support Liver Health

Dietary balance and nutrient richness are the keys to supporting your liver as well as healthy weight loss.

Because both processes rely on the same dietary foundation of nourishment, good balance and nutrient-richness work equally well for weight loss and liver health.

The World's Healthiest Foods are essential for providing your liver with a concentrated and diverse mixture of metabolic-support nutrients. If you can choose the certified organic version of nutrient-rich World's Healthiest Foods, you can avoid unnecessary metabolic loads on your liver caused by toxic residues found in non-organic foods (for more on organic foods, see page 199). Because the World's Healthiest Foods are minimally processed, they benefit liver health by relieving your liver of the task of processing additives. An approach to food that emphasizes the aforementioned principles—relying on nutrient-rich World's Healthiest Foods as the foundation of your diet, and choosing organically grown varieties whenever possible—can work wonders for your liver and keep your weight loss process healthy.

What is the significance of the liver in healthy weight loss? Losing weight takes a toll on our bodies from a metabolic standpoint. It is a metabolic challenge for our bodies to transition from weight maintenance to weight loss. Along with the digestive tract, our liver is at the heart of this process. In terms of metabolism, our liver is where things get sorted out. A healthy liver is required for both the breakdown of fat into energy and the transport of unwanted fat.

Production of energy to fuel the brain during times of metabolic stress is also affected. A healthy liver is required for healthy blood sugar balance, wakefulness and sleep, and vitamin and mineral processing.

Will you feel well enough to continue your weight loss efforts? Will you be able to maintain the process for many months because you feel healthy and capable? The answers to those questions directly point to your liver as the organ system responsible for metabolic challenges and optimal metabolism. As you can see, supporting your liver is a critical aspect of encouraging healthy weight loss, and the World's Healthiest Foods contain nutrients that can promote liver health.

CHAPTER EIGHT

The World's Healthiest Foods Maintain Blood Sugar Balance

Maintaining Blood Sugar Balance

Glucose, a type of sugar found in our blood, is essential for many cells, particularly the brain. Having balanced blood glucose levels is an important aspect of staying healthy. Our cells may not be properly nourished if these levels are too low. If these levels are too high, metabolic consequences can occur, causing kidney, artery, and other body system damage. High blood glucose levels usually indicate that the cells are unable to absorb glucose and thus do not receive the energy required for normal function.

When we talk about blood sugar, we are not referring to the same type of sugar that is found in table sugar. Blood sugar is glucose, a simple sugar that can be broken down into other sugars.

Our blood sugar levels fluctuate slightly throughout the day. Eating a meal can significantly alter our blood sugar levels, depending on the foods we eat and how thoroughly we chew and digest them. It is normal for our blood sugar to rise after eating. However, it is unnatural for it to exceed certain limits. Similarly, it is natural for our blood sugar to drop between meals. Excessive drops, on the other hand, are a problem.

If we eat in a way that causes our blood sugar balance to fluctuate, we risk several negative consequences, including the possibility of weight gain. The link between large blood sugar swings and potential weight gain is straightforward. If our blood sugar rises dramatically and then falls, we may perceive the drop as a need for more food to raise our blood sugar back up to its elevated level. Similarly, if we go too long without eating and our blood sugar "bottoms out" at an abnormally low level, we may feel desperate for anything. The rollercoaster ride can be dangerous for overeating in either direction.

When our blood sugar swings dramatically, we are more likely to crave high-sugar, high-calorie, and nutrient-deficient foods. This situation can only increase our chances of gaining weight.

Processed foods high in simple sugar will spike our blood sugar faster than whole, natural foods. These processed foods are frequently high in refined carbohydrates, almost never contain enough fiber to balance digestion and allow for a slow breakdown and release of carbohydrates into our digestive tract, and are frequently deficient in the vitamins and minerals required to support insulin production and glucose uptake into our cells. This can cause a yo-yo effect in our blood sugar levels and increase our chances of gaining weight.

The World's Healthiest Foods are high in vitamins, minerals, fiber, and other health-promoting compounds that can assist us in maintaining optimal blood sugar regulation. They are high in fiber, which helps to slow digestion. They contain chromium and vitamin B3, both of which are involved in the process of insulin metabolism and the hormone's ability to remove sugar from our bloodstream.

Many of the World's Healthiest Foods are also high in zinc, a mineral that helps regulate blood sugar levels.

So you can see how eating nutrient-dense World's Healthiest Foods can help you maintain a healthy blood sugar level. This nutrient contribution will not only help you lose weight, but it will also provide you with significant overall health benefits because high blood sugar levels can lead to insulin resistance, which is now recognized as a critical factor in the development of many health conditions.

Insulin Deficiency
Health scientists have long regarded the development of a chronic disease, such as obesity, diabetes, or high blood pressure, as a complex process involving numerous factors. Insulin resistance is one of the most prominent factors in this mix. Over 900 research studies focused solely on insulin resistance and its relationship to long-term health in 2007. Insulin resistance has become so

central to our understanding of health that it is no longer possible to comprehend a seemingly simple process such as chronic weight gain without considering insulin resistance and its potential role in the process.

The Causes of Insulin Resistance:

Sugar is the most common source of energy in our bodies (glucose.)

When our cells require energy, sugar is the most commonly used fuel. Sugar, which our cells require, is constantly flowing through our blood. However, in order for sugar to leave our bloodstream and enter our cells, insulin—a protein hormone produced by our pancreas— is usually required. Insulin resistance occurs when this process fails and our cells stop responding effectively to the insulin produced by our pancreas. In order to get sugar into our cells, our pancreas may produce an unusually large amount of insulin. However, insulin resistance prevents this effort from being fully effective because insulin's actions are still being resisted in some way. The term "insulin resistance" refers to this unfavorable set of events. Insulin resistance can become more than just a temporary stumbling block to health.

How Insulin Resistance Affects Weight Management: The relationship between insulin resistance and body weight is not simple or straightforward. However, there are a few distinguishing characteristics. For starters, excess body weight in the form of excess fat—particularly around the middle (or abdomen)—is linked to the development of insulin resistance. Insulin resistance is significantly more likely to occur in men with waist circumferences greater than 40 inches and in women with waist circumferences greater than 35 inches.

How does extra abdominal fat contribute to insulin resistance?

This sequence of events is not entirely clear to researchers. Traditionally, all insulin and blood sugar balance research has focused on muscle rather than fat. When insulin assists sugar in leaving the bloodstream, it usually assists sugar in entering a muscle cell rather than a fat cell.

Because muscles are so important in receiving sugar from the blood, the role of fat cells in blood sugar balance has been overlooked until recently. However, recent research has revealed that fat cells (also known as adipose tissue) play an important role in insulin metabolism and blood sugar regulation. One of these links, as described in the chapter on inflammation, is related to the fact that overly fatty fat cells produce insufficient amounts of adiponectin, a protein that assists insulin in locking onto cells and escorting sugar out of our blood. When adiponectin levels are low, too much sugar remains in the blood, causing our pancreas to produce more insulin to compensate. More insulin, however, will not solve the real problem. The true issue is insulin resistance, which in this case is caused by too much abdominal body fat.

Insulin Resistance and the Proclivity to Gain Weight:

Just as excess abdominal fat can increase our proclivity to develop insulin resistance, insulin resistance can increase our proclivity to gain weight. Insulin resistance increases the risk of weight gain and obesity, especially in women who are lean and have lower levels of total body fat. Women who have gone through menopause are also more likely to gain weight as a result of the development of insulin resistance. However, in obese women, insulin resistance may actually protect against weight gain and make weight loss easier. Finally, there is some intriguing research indicating that people who develop insulin resistance while also getting a high percentage of their total calories from fat have a higher risk of gaining weight and becoming obese than people who have insulin resistance but only get a moderate percentage of their total calories from fat.

How the World's Healthiest Foods Can Aid in the Prevention of Insulin Resistance and Weight Gain

There are three basic ways that your diet can aid in the prevention of insulin resistance. Fortunately, the World's Healthiest Foods can help you in all three of these areas.

The first task is to avoid or eliminate excess abdominal fat.

(If you are already overweight and have excess fat around your midsection, you will want to avoid adding more abdominal fat.) Because the risk of insulin resistance increases as the amount of abdominal fat increases, this step appears to be critical. Even if you already have too much fat around your middle, or if your waistline is fine and you're just trying to avoid unwanted weight gain around your middle, you'll want to prioritize the World's Healthiest Foods in your diet because they are the key to reduced risk of insulin resistance. Even though there is no way to "spot reduce" and lose fat pounds only from your midsection, overall weight loss will include fat loss from your midsection, and you can achieve this overall weight loss most effectively with nutrient-rich World's Healthiest Foods.

The second task is to avoid a high-fat diet. People who develop insulin resistance and consume a high percentage of their total calories from fat are more likely to gain weight than those who develop insulin resistance but consume only a moderate percentage of their total calories from fat. As you can see, the menus in the Healthy Weight Loss Eating Plan contain an average of 249 total calories from fat. This is ideal for limiting fat intake and lowering the risk of weight gain due to insulin resistance.

The third, and perhaps most important, goal is to keep your blood sugar as stable as possible through diet. The World's Healthiest Foods listed here can help you in a variety of ways. Because they help regulate the rate of digestion, high-fiber foods are essential for blood sugar stabilization. And because the majority of the World's Healthiest Foods are plant-based, they are naturally high in fiber.

Protein-rich foods are also important for blood sugar control.

Protein digests slowly, which is good for blood sugar levels.

Rich protein sources include lean meats, fish, low-fat dairy foods, legumes, and the majority of the nuts and seeds on the World's Healthiest Foods list.

Finally, nothing is more damaging to our blood sugar levels than a diet high in processed foods that have had the fiber, vitamins, and minerals removed. Because the Healthy Weight Loss - Without Dieting program emphasizes the World's Healthiest Foods, it keeps these processed foods out of your regular meal plan, which pays huge dividends in terms of blood sugar balance.

Choosing Foods Based on the Glycemic Index to Maintain Balanced Blood Sugar Levels

It's important to remember that not all foods, even the World's Healthiest Foods, are created equal in terms of their effects on our blood sugar levels. Some foods cause sharp spikes in blood sugar levels, while others keep them relatively stable.

The Glycemic Index (GI) is a numerical scale that indicates how quickly and how significantly a specific food can raise our blood glucose (blood sugar) level. A low GI food will typically cause a moderate rise in blood glucose, whereas a high GI food may cause our blood glucose level to rise above the optimal level.

Choosing foods based on their GI is an excellent way to manage blood sugar fluctuations.

An understanding of the GI of foods can help you control your blood sugar levels, which can help you achieve or maintain a healthy weight, as well as prevent heart disease, improve cholesterol levels, and prevent insulin resistance, type 2 diabetes, and certain cancers. A substantial amount of research indicates that a low-GI diet provides these significant health benefits and can be an important component of a healthy weight loss strategy.

CHAPTER NINE

The World's Healthiest Foods Lower Inflammation

In this chapter, I'd like to introduce you to a new area of medical research: the role of inflammation in healthy weight loss. Although my main focus will be on inflammation, I will also tell you about your fat-burning processes and how to avoid certain problems in these areas.

What exactly is inflammation?
These days, we hear a lot about inflammation and how it contributes to health conditions like cardiovascular disease and arthritis.

Before I get into the link between inflammation and weight loss, I wanted to define inflammation.

Inflammation is a normal biological reaction that occurs in the body. Inflammation in general is not a bad thing, and we don't want to stop all inflammatory mechanisms in our bodies if we want to promote good health. What we want to do is control inflammation and prevent excessive inflammation in our bodies. It is imbalanced inflammation that can cause health conditions and symptoms, as well as play a role in weight management.

Fat Storage Cell Reduction and Inflammation Control

In the last decade, the study of fat cells and their role in health has yielded some surprising results, including the discovery that fat cells are anything but inactive fat storage spots. We're used to thinking of body fat as "just sitting there," putting extra weight on our bones and putting strain on our hearts and joints from the extra poundage.

In the last ten years, we've learned that fat cells are metabolically active, and when there's too much fat stored inside them, they go to work sending messages that increase inflammation and inflammatory problems. Some of the signaling molecules that indicate inflammation are only produced in excessively fatty fat cells! Fat cells, on the other hand, can produce anti-inflammatory molecules, and the production of these molecules can be reduced when the fat cells become overloaded with fat.

Understanding Leptin and Fat Cells

Leptin is a particularly important molecule produced by our fat cells.

When we have insufficient fat stored in our fat cells, our fat cells reduce their production of leptin.

When we overeat and our fat stores become too large, the opposite set of events occurs. Under these conditions, our fat cells begin to produce an increasing amount of leptin. The increased production of leptin will, in turn, cause two sets of events: it will reduce our appetite and increase our body's ability to burn fat.

At this point in the narrative, we've arrived at the role of inflammation.

It turns out that most people who have an excess of fat stored in their fat cells also have an abundance of leptin. Their fat cells appear to do a good job of increasing leptin production when this molecule is required to help lower appetite and increase fat burning.

Despite this abundant supply of leptin, the leptin does not appear to be doing its job effectively. Even though more leptin is produced, appetite suppression and increased fat burn do not appear to occur. Leptin resistance refers to this clearly problematic situation. Our bodies appear to resist the effects of leptin, despite the fact that they would benefit greatly if leptin could do its job.

According to research, inflammation is one factor that can contribute to leptin resistance. In fact, it may be the primary cause of leptin resistance in many people. Although it is unclear how the two are linked, people who have chronic, low-grade inflammation are more likely to develop leptin resistance. Anyone who lives or eats in a way that increases their risk of chronic, unwanted inflammation is also increasing their risk of appetite and fat-burning issues due to leptin resistance. This set of facts is one clear reason why the Healthiest Way of Eating includes a significant amount of anti-inflammatory foods.

Adiponectin Can Influence Weight Loss

Adiponectin, like leptin, is a regulatory molecule produced by our fat cells. Unlike leptin, however, adiponectin is produced in lower (rather than higher) quantities by our fat cells when we overeat and begin storing too much unwanted body fat. Adiponectin functions as a "fat protector," ensuring that enough fat is available during times of low energy supply. Excessive and continuous overeating, on the other hand, leads to chronic adiponectin deficiency, which is harmful rather than beneficial to our health.

Adiponectin is a fat-cell-produced anti-inflammatory molecule that suffers when fat cells become overloaded with fat.

When adiponectin production falls, so does the body's ability to balance blood sugar. The reason is straightforward. Adiponectin, a protein produced by fat cells, aids in the binding of insulin to cells and promotes the flow of sugar from the bloodstream into the cells. When fat cells stop producing enough adiponectin, there is an excess of sugar in the blood.

Managing Inflammation

What does this complicated series of events mean for a meal plan based on the World's Healthiest Foods? For starters, it implies that a diet that prevents fat accumulation in fat cells is highly desirable. Which diet best prevents fat accumulation in fat cells? According to research, it is the diet that contains the highest percentage of nutrient-rich foods, such as the World's Healthiest Foods—foods that provide the greatest variety and quantity of nutrients for the fewest calories. Second, when there is a weight problem, blood sugar balance and inflammatory balance are critical. Because the World's Healthiest Foods are high in nutrients that are necessary for blood sugar regulation, insulin regulation, and inflammatory balance, they are also your best bet if you have excess fat in your fat cells. They are the ideal foods for safely transporting you from here (excess fat in fat cells) to there (fat cells that do not trigger inflammation due to excess fat storage).

I believe that avoiding chronic inflammation is critical for weight management. When the body is inflamed, it not only risks damaging cells and tissues and causing a domino-like cascade that can lead to disease, but it also depletes our nutrient reserves. It will seek antioxidant and anti-inflammatory nutrients to help prevent unfavorable physiological events. This process, in turn, reduces the supply of nutrients available to our bodies for other functions.

Remember that inflammation can disrupt our fat cells' metabolism and the communication that our fat cells are attempting to have with our brain, digestive system, and bloodstream. Inflammation can present us with a new food-related risk by disrupting our fat cell metabolism. This risk is unrelated to any temptations we may experience. It's a risk of overeating that stems from disruption in the control of our appetite and control of our fat burning processes.

Whether you are trying to lose weight, maintain a recent weight loss, or healthfully maintain the ideal weight you have been at for a while, it pays to stay well nourished in a way that allows your metabolism to adjust along with your new or changing weight. You will be short-changing your metabolism if you drain too many nutrient resources while trying to cope with chronic inflammation.

The last few years of research about inflammation and obesity make me more convinced than ever about the value of the World's Healthiest Foods! I have always believed that nutrient-richness was a key to successful weight loss. How could a person possibly go through a challenging period of time like weight loss without needing more nutritional support for their body's metabolism? The answer is: they couldn't! But how could a person get more nutritional support at a time when they clearly needed to eat less food? The answer nutrient-richness—pack more nourishment in fewer calories.

Now research studies have given us the added issue of inflammation.

They have told us that inflammation is the part of obesity that can lead to diabetes and heart disease. Inflammation is the part of obesity that can even lead to premature death. This new set of discoveries about inflammation has made us realize what's really at stake when we are trying to lose weight. When we undertake the weight loss process, we are not only trying to lower some numbers on the scale or fit back into old clothes. We are also trying to prevent our bodies from becoming metabolically out-of-balance in a potentially permanent way that will go far beyond the presence of unwanted fat around our middle.

The obesity-inflammation research has made me realize how important the nutrient-rich anti-inflammatory diet—an approach to eating that will prevent the occurrence of unwanted inflammation and avoid that slippery slope between obesity and diabetes and heart disease—really is. But what's most exciting for me to report is the ability of the World's Healthiest Foods to accomplish both tasks at once. The same foods that provide you with the highest forms of nutrient-richness simultaneously provide you with the very best anti-inflammatory nutrients. These nutrients include omega-3 fatty acids, many vitamins and minerals, flavonoids, carotenoids, and a long list of other phytonutrients that are unsurpassed in other foods. Read on to learn more about these health-promoting nutrients.

Food Choices Can Help Prevent Inflammation
Always keep in mind that what you eat can help with inflammation in three different ways. These three aspects are taken into consideration in the Healthy Weight Loss Eating Plan, which will show you examples of how to construct a nutrient-rich way of eating that helps to keep inflammation in check.

First, what you eat can be adjusted to avoid deficiency of anti-inflammatory nutrients. An inadequate supply of omega-3 fatty acids, for example, can increase the risk of chronic inflammation.

By adjusting the diet to include more omega-3s, the risk of chronic inflammation can be lowered.

Second, what you eat can be adjusted to avoid triggering too much inflammation. Since toxins found in food can serve as inflammatory triggers, you can lower your risk of unwanted and chronic inflammation by eliminating these toxins from your meal plan as much as possible

Finally, a diet can be adjusted to avoid imbalances that trigger chronic inflammation. A diet that contains too many processed foods, for example, will provide too many calories in the form of simple sugars and too few calories from nutrient-rich foods. By shifting the balance in this area, unwanted inflammation can become less likely. Let's look at some basic dos and don'ts in each of these three areas.

Getting Plenty of Anti-Inflammatory Nutrients

At the top of the list for anti-inflammatory nutrients are two broad groups of phytonutrients called flavonoids and carotenoids. Many flavonoids and carotenoids have potent anti-inflammatory properties that are often specific to the food in question. Richly colored vegetables and fruits are some of your best bets here, including dark green leafy vegetables, beets, and berries. Pineapple also contains bromclain, a proteolytic (protein-digesting) enzyme that has been shown to have anti-inflammatory activity. These foods are included among the World's Healthiest Foods.

Some studies have found that people who consume a lot of flavonoids and carotenoids do not have a lower risk of chronic inflammation. These studies make it clear that there are no "magic bullets" when it comes to dietary prevention of chronic disease. While it's important to ensure that you are getting adequate supplies of carotenoids and flavonoids, this shouldn't be at the expense of other nutrients, since all are important. Yet, luckily since carotenoid- and flavonoid-containing foods are also generally rich in so many other vitamins and minerals, they can make great overall contributions to your nutrient goals.

Foods rich in omega-3 fatty acids can also be considered anti-inflammatory because omega-3 fatty acids like alpha-linolenic acid (ALA), eicosapentaenoic acid (EPA), and docosahexaenoic acid (DHA) can be converted into regulatory molecules that put the brakes on inflammation. Foods rich in omega-3 fatty acids include: fish such as salmon, sardines, tuna, and other cold-water fish; and, nuts and seeds, especially flaxseeds, hemp seeds, and walnuts. Other foods that contain omega-3s in lesser, but still very helpful, amounts include soybeans, winter squash, and purslane.

Extra virgin olive oil is another food that has been shown to have anti-inflammatory benefits. Some of these benefits come from oleuropein and hydroxytyrosol, two unique polyphenols found in olives.

It is important to note that these two phytonutrients are more concentrated in extra virgin olive than in other types of olive oil. As you'll see in the Healthy Weight Loss Eating Plan, I place a strong emphasis on extra virgin olive oil because it has such great health benefits.

Avoiding Inflammatory Triggers in Your Meal Plan

Artificial additives, including colors, flavors, and preservatives can all trigger unwanted inflammatory response in the body, not only in the digestive system, but in other body systems once these food toxins get absorbed. On a day-in and day-out basis, processed foods containing these additives can trigger chronic, low-level inflammation throughout the body. The Healthy Weight Loss Eating Plan avoid these inflammatory triggers.

To lower your risk in this area, your best bet is to choose whole foods that are organically grown whenever possible. Locally grown, seasonal foods are also usually lower in total toxins because they have undergone processing and don't require the same kind of preservation for extended shelf life. If you cannot purchase either organic or seasonal, locally grown foods, fresh whole foods—like fresh fruits and vegetables in their whole, natural form—are still likely to be lower in total toxins than processed foods found in pre-packaged frozen dinners or other pre-packaged items.

Achieving a Dietary Balance That Will Prevent Unwanted Inflammation

Overall dietary balance (and lifestyle balance as well) is extremely important in preventing chronic inflammation. It's impossible for any nutrient, or even a large group of nutrients, to overcome the problems associated with an unbalanced diet. If your diet includes too much fat (especially long chain saturated fat), too many processed foods with simple sugars and little fiber, inadequate protein, too many calories, too few calories, poor timing, or poor eating habits (like inadequate chewing and eating under stress), it is going to be impossible for your anti-inflammatory nutrients to do their job.

This same word of caution applies to lifestyle. Multiple studies show the powerful role of regular exercise in reducing risk of chronic inflammation. Healthy and adequate sleep is also clearly documented as an important component of an anti-inflammatory lifestyle. Don't count on your diet alone to offset a long list of imbalanced living habits.

Maintaining an Anti-Inflammatory Diet

I want you to know that the inflammation story is far from over, and you can expect to see a lot of new research in this area, including weight loss research. Some of the most intriguing research may be in the field of cells and their development.

Many scientists already believe that some of our cells go through a kind of decision point where they must choose whether to become fat cells or another type of cell called macrophages. Macrophages are white blood cell-derived cells that play an important role in our body's immune system. Their name is derived from the Greek words makros, which means "large," and phagein, which means "to eat." As "big eaters," macrophages are designed to assist our bodies in eliminating potentially harmful substances and microorganisms.

Macrophages may make up nearly half of the cells found in fat tissue (adipose tissue) in some people. This close relationship between our fat cells and our immune system is likely to provide us with a new understanding of the events involved in excess fat storage as well as fat loss.

Aside from the inflammation issue, there is a general recognition that weight loss is more than just counting calories. It also has to do with our physiological health, the metabolic regulation of our appetite, fat burning processes, and other aspects of our metabolism. I don't think future research will ever "let us off the hook" in terms of calories, temptations, and other all-too-familiar aspects of weight loss. But I expect it to introduce new variables into the mix and provide us with novel and unexpected ways to succeed in this aspect of our health!

SECTION 3

The Eating Plan for Healthy Weight Loss

CHAPTER TEN

The Eating Plan for Healthy Weight Loss

Introduction

What exactly is a Healthy Weight Loss Eating Plan?
The Healthy Weight Loss Eating Plan was created to provide you with nutritious meals that are also delicious.

your taste buds, satisfying in terms of amount, and make weight loss an attainable goal. The Plan's four weeks of menus were designed to provide you with a basic blueprint—a practical guideline for weight loss. What I hope is that you can use the 4-week blueprint as a starting point for developing your own personalized strategy for long-term healthy weight loss.

Who will benefit from the Plan's implementation:
The Plan was created to improve the health of the average person who is overweight and wants to become healthier through healthy weight loss. The Plan is not a clinical plan, nor is it intended to address clinical issues. If you have any clinical issues in your healthcare, including any that may impact your choice of a weight loss plan, you should seek the assistance of your healthcare provider. In general, because our weight loss plan contains approximately 1,530 calories per day, we

anticipate that it will provide the greatest weight loss benefit to individuals who are currently consuming a significantly higher level of calories.

Before implementing the Plan, who should consult a healthcare practitioner:

Before beginning our weight loss program, the following people should consult with their healthcare provider:

• All pregnant women, women who are nursing, and women who are considering becoming pregnant

• All individuals under 18 years of age

• All individuals who are concerned about obtaining Daily Value levels of nutrient intake for all nutrients based on diet alone and without the help of dietary supplements.

• All individuals with special concerns about their intake of vitamin D, vitamin B5, vitamin B12, or zinc.

What to Expect When Following the Plan:

In the United States, adults consume approximately 2,100 calories per day. Adults in the United States are, on average, overweight, and their calorie intake is related to their weight status. Because our weight loss plan averages about 1,530 calories per day, it represents a daily reduction of about 570 calories for the average adult in the United States. That 570-calorie-per-day reduction would be expected to result in a weight loss of about 1 pound over a week if all other factors remained constant. The expected weight loss in one month is 4 pounds, and 48 pounds in one year.

Whatever weight loss plan you use, your daily calorie intake must be properly matched to your activity level. You can expect to maintain your current weight if you consume exactly the number of daily calories required to complete your daily activities (including exercise). You can expect to gain weight if you exceed that number. You can expect to lose weight if you consume fewer calories than are required to complete your daily activities (including exercise). Of course, in practice, weight loss never occurs with such mathematical precision!

The number of calories expended by exercising is determined by personal factors such as body weight. There are numerous calorie expenditure calculators available on the Internet that you can use to calculate how many calories you will burn by participating in various types of exercise and activities.

Remember, before beginning any exercise program, consult with your doctor, who should be familiar enough with your health to provide you with personalized guidelines and any important do's and don'ts.

When you follow the Plan, you can expect to develop a sense of foods, food groups, food selection, recipes, and menu planning that can serve as a springboard for developing your own ongoing weight loss approach that takes advantage of nutrient-rich, whole natural foods and fits with your individual health status and lifestyle. You should also get a sense of how a healthy 1,530 calorie diet feels and how it fits in with your other lifestyle goals. Many people will not be able to see weekly changes in their weight status on a 1,530-calorie diet unless they incorporate daily exercise into their weight loss plan.

How to Begin the Plan:

Welcome to the Healthy Weight Loss Eating Plan, a 28-day guide to weight loss. I believe that anyone can live a healthy lifestyle and be slim, and that eating healthier has an impact on how you feel, how much energy you have, and how healthy you are. I've devised a comprehensive plan to help you lose weight, regain control of your health, boost your immune system, and rejuvenate your entire body. This Plan will introduce you to some of the most nutritious foods available—The World's Healthiest Foods.

While you will most likely feel the benefits in the first few days, it takes about 4 weeks for a habit to become established. So, give yourself this time and be patient with yourself as you begin this journey.

Journey to the Healthiest Way of Eating: The Plan is not a diet or an expensive, time-consuming program.

It is a method of starting a lifestyle change toward the Healthiest Way of Eating.

And I've done all of the legwork for you, so it's simple! I offer recipes that not only taste great but also take only minutes to prepare—most take 7 minutes or less, and you can make an entire meal in 15 minutes! You only need to go shopping, and you won't have to break the bank to get the ingredients for these recipes.

The Advantages of the Healthy Weight Loss Eating Plan:

The plan includes 28 days of daily menus that promote the Healthiest Way of Eating. Because each of the week's breakfasts, lunches, dinners, and snacks have a similar level of calories and nutrients, the Plan includes a flexible approach that allows you to swap meals from one day to the next if desired. This will allow you to tailor the Plan to your specific requirements.

- **Healthier Lifestyle Tea:**

The Plan includes a cup of Healthier Lifestyle Tea to drink before each meal. Green tea and lemon juice are used to make this tea. Green tea is not only tasty, but it is also known for its health-promoting properties. These have been linked to a high concentration of catechin phytonutrients, which have numerous protective benefits, many of which are related to their potent ability to cleanse free radicals.

Adding 1 teaspoon lemon juice to each cup of green tea not only adds a refreshing flavor but also provides additional benefits. There have been studies that show that drinking green tea can help you lose weight; for example, in one study, participants lost 5% of their body weight and circumference in three months. Drink decaffeinated green tea if you are sensitive to caffeine or want to limit your caffeine intake.

- **High-Energy Breakfast:**

Breakfasts contain good carbohydrates, primarily from fruits and whole grains, as well as delicious protein-rich foods, primarily from nuts, seeds, and eggs, to provide you with the energy you need to get through the morning feeling satisfied and to curb your appetite until lunch. They provide omega-3 fatty acids from walnuts and flaxseeds. Their appetite-satisfying properties are also due to the high levels of dietary fiber they contain.

Snack to energize you.

Every day, you'll enjoy energizing snacks with delectable flavors. Sweet fruits will satisfy your sweet tooth while also providing you with vitamins, minerals, phytonutrients, and other nutrients. Nuts and seeds provide protein and other nutrients that may help reduce blood sugar fluctuations. According to studies, people who eat nuts and seeds in moderation tend to be slimmer than those who don't eat these delicious foods.

- **Power Lunch:**

The Plan's lunches are delicious and fill your stomach. They contain a good balance of protein, carbohydrates, and healthy fats.

Most lunches include a delicious salad, which is an important aspect of a healthy weight loss strategy. For example, one study discovered that women who ate a large low-calorie salad ate 12% less pasta even when given unlimited amounts. Not only will your appetite be satisfied, but you'll also benefit greatly from all of the important nutrients it contains. According to studies, people who ate one large salad with dressing per day had higher levels of vitamin C and E, folic acid, lycopene, and other carotenoids than those who did not include salad in their daily diet. All of this without consuming a lot of calories; for example, 2 cups of romaine lettuce could be used as the base of a salad. This salad green has a delicious flavor and satisfying crunch, as well as a plethora of vitamins, minerals, phytonutrients, antioxidants, and fiber. It also has only 16 calories. Salads suppress your appetite, allowing you to consume fewer calories over the course of a meal.

Legumes and beans are also highlighted in some of the lunches. Because these foods are so slow to digest, many people regard them as natural appetite suppressants. With their low glycemic index (GI) they keep blood sugar on an even keel and stave off hunger.

Good fats, such as omega-3s found in seafood and monounsaturated fats found in extra virgin olive oil, are beneficial to health on multiple levels, including aiding in the absorption of fat-soluble nutrients and phytonutrients. Extra virgin olive oil is a concentrated source of monounsaturated fats that has antioxidant nutrients and also helps to enhance the flavor of the dishes to which it is applied.

According to some studies, extra virgin olive oil can cause a small but significant loss of body weight and mass.

- **Slimming Dinner:**

Each dinner begins with an Appetizer Satisfier of crudite vegetables. This will assist you in not overeating and feeling satisfied. And keep you from going hungry while you're cooking dinner.

Let me share with you one of my favorite quick-and-easy Appetizer Satisfiers. I tear a few leaves from a head of romaine lettuce, wash them, shake off the water, and sprinkle with salt before eating. (When using the outer big leaves, I cut off the tips because they can be bitter and dry). The ancient Romans were known to eat this salted lettuce; in fact, the word salad is derived from their name for this salted lettuce—salata.

The foods featured are also high in fiber, which helps to suppress appetite and improve digestion. Many herbs and spices, such as ginger, cayenne pepper, turmeric, mustard, and garlic, are used in the dinner recipes. They not only add flavor, but they are also high in nutrients, including those that promote healthy digestion. Because the dinners are filling but not too heavy, they may also help you sleep better.

Each dinner comes with a Green Power Side Dish. These simple-to-prepare foods are the foundation of the Healthiest Way of Eating.

These foods are high in chlorophyll and contain a variety of nutrients (including flavonoid and carotenoid antioxidants), but they are low in calories, making them essential for healthy weight loss. These nutrients will help support optimal metabolism because they provide the nutrients your body systems require; if you don't have enough nutrients to support your metabolism, you won't be able to optimize your weight loss.

Green Power Side Dishes can be extremely beneficial for healthy weight loss. Consider that eating two cups of green vegetables instead of a baked potato with butter or margarine will save you over 300 calories. These foods are also low in GI, which aids in blood sugar regulation.

- **Sweet Desserts:**

While desserts are not required in the Plan, I believe that fresh fruit is a great option because it can satisfy a sweet tooth while also providing a wealth of health-promoting nutrients. These nutrients contain antioxidants, which help to neutralize free radicals in the body. When it comes to weight loss, choosing a healthy sweet dessert can really make a difference; for example, a parfait made with low-fat yogurt and berries will save you 200 calories compared to eating one cup of ice cream.

The Healthy Weight Loss Eating Plan
Week 1

Week 1 (Day 1)

This day of the Healthy Weight Loss Eating Plan includes easy-to-prepare menus with exciting flavors and good nutrition; you'll have plenty of delicious foods to keep you satisfied. High-fiber cereal with fruit and nuts for the High-Energy Breakfast, a Mediterranean Caesar Salad for the Power Lunch, and tasty salmon with Dill Sauce over Spinach for the Slimming Dinner. You'll also get a High-Energy Snack of apple, almond butter, orange, and walnuts; an Appetizer Satisfier of crudite and guacamole; a Green Power Side Dish of broccoli; and Healthier Lifestyle Tea. These meals are made up of nutrient-dense foods that provide you with many of the health-promoting nutrients you require on a daily basis.

Breakfast

1 cup fiber-rich cereal

½ cup fresh blueberries

2 tablespoons chopped walnuts

1 sliced banana

1 cup skim non-fat milk

Snack for Energy:

1 apple, medium size

1 tablespoon almond butter

Lunch

Mediterranean Caesar Salad

Snack for Energy:

1 orange, medium-sized

three walnut halves

Dinner

Appetizer:

1 cup carrot slices/strips

1 celery stick cup

1 cup cucumber slices

Guacamole in 3 Minutes

Week 1 (Day 2)

This day of the Healthy Weight Loss Eating Plan includes easy-to-prepare menus with exciting flavors and good nutrition; you'll have plenty of delicious foods to keep you satisfied. A Tropical Energy Smoothie will be served for the High-Energy Breakfast, a Mediterranean Turkey Salad with Mushrooms for the Power Lunch, and a tasty Mediterranean Cod with Red Peppers and Basil for the Slimming Dinner. You'll also get a High-Energy Snack of pears, almonds, and grapes; an Appetizer Satisfier of zucchini, carrots, and cauliflower; a Green Power Side Dish with kale; and a Healthier Lifestyle Tea. These meals are made up of nutrient-dense foods that provide you with many of the health-promoting nutrients you require on a daily basis.

Breakfast

Tropical Energy Smoothie high-energy breakfast

Energizing snack:

1 medium-sized pear

3 almonds

Lunch

Mediterranean Turkey Salad with Mushrooms

Energizing Snack:

1 cup red grapes

3 almonds

Dinner

Appetizers:

1 cup sliced zucchini

½ cup carrots, sliced

½ cup florets cauliflower

Cod with Red Peppers and Basil from the Mediterranean

Mashed Sweet Potatoes

Week 1 (Day 3)

This day of the Healthy Weight Loss Eating Plan includes easy-to-prepare menus with exciting flavors and good nutrition; you'll have plenty of delicious foods to keep you satisfied. Poached egg with Swiss chard for the High-Energy Breakfast, Romaine Salad with Goat Cheese and Mushrooms for the Power Lunch, and Spicy Asian Shrimp with Spinach for the Slimming Dinner. You'll also get a High-Energy Snack of papaya, walnuts, pear, and almonds; an Appetizer Satisfier of bell peppers, carrots, and cucumber; a Green Power Side Dish of broccoli; and a Healthier Lifestyle Tea. These meals are made up of nutrient-dense foods that provide you with many of the health-promoting nutrients you require on a daily basis.

Tea for a Healthier Lifestyle

Breakfast

3 minutes Swiss chard 2 topped with 1/4 cup pumpkin seeds, 1 tablespoon sunflower seeds, and 1 poached egg.

1 whole wheat toast slice

½ cantaloupes

Energizing Snack:

3 walnut halves

papaya with lime

Lunch

Salad with Goat Cheese and Mushrooms

Energizing Snack:

3 pears and 3 almonds

Dinner

Appetizer:

½ cup red bell peppers, sliced

½ cup carrot sticks/slices

½ cup sliced cucumber

Spicy Asian Shrimp served with rice

Side Dish:

1-minute spinach, 3 minutes broccoli, and 1 tablespoon sunflower seeds.

Week 1 (Day 4)

This day of the Healthy Weight Loss Eating Plan includes easy-to-prepare menus with exciting flavors and good nutrition; you'll have plenty of delicious foods to keep you satisfied. Yogurt with fruit for the High-Energy Breakfast, Greek Salad with Garbanzo Beans and Feta Cheese for the Power Lunch, and Salmon with Ginger Mint Salsa for the Slimming Dinner. You'll also get a High-Energy Snack of orange, Brazil nuts, figs, and almonds; an Appetizer Satisfier of cucumbers, bell peppers, and zucchini; a Green Power Side Dish with Swiss chard; and a Healthier Lifestyle Tea. These meals are made up of nutrient-dense foods that provide you with many of the health-promoting nutrients you require on a daily basis.

Breakfast

1 tbsp blackstrap molasses in 8 oz cup plain non-fat yogurt

½ cup fresh blueberries

½ large fresh papaya

1 banana, medium

1 whole wheat toast slice

Snack for Energy:

1 orange, medium size

1 nut of Brazil

Lunch

Salad with Garbanzo Beans and Feta from Greece.

Energizing Snack:

2 dried figs

3 dried almonds

Dinner

Appetizer:

1 celery stick cup

1 cup sliced cucumber

1 cup carrot sticks or slices

Guacamole Salmon with Ginger Mint Salsa on top.

Week 1 (Day 5)

This day of the Healthy Weight Loss Eating Plan includes easy-to-prepare menus with exciting flavors and good nutrition; you'll have plenty of delicious foods to keep you satisfied. Poached Egg over Spinach and Mushrooms for the High-Energy Breakfast, Healthy Chef's Salad with Cheddar Cheese and Garbanzo Beans for the Power Lunch, and Halibut with Ginger and Scallions for the Slimming Dinner. You'll also get a High-Energy Snack of apple, sunflower seeds, orange segments, and almonds; an Appetizer Satisfier of bell peppers, cucumbers, and carrots; a Green Power Side Dish with Brussels sprouts, and Healthier Lifestyle Tea. These meals are made up of nutrient-dense foods that provide you with many of the health-promoting nutrients you require on a daily basis.

Breakfast

Combine 1-Minute Spinach 1 with Healthy Sautéed Crimini Mushrooms for a High-Energy Breakfast. 2 tops with 1 poached egg on top, preferably an omega-rich egg.

1 whole wheat toast slice

½ cantaloupes

Energizing Snack:

1 medium apple and 6 almonds

Lunch

Healthy Chef's Salad with Cheddar Cheese and Garbanzo Beans.

Energizing Snack:

1 medium orange and 6 almonds

Dinner

Appetizer:

½ cup red bell peppers, sliced

½ cup cucumber slices

½ cup carrot sticks/slices

Halibut with Scallions and Ginger

Cauliflower with Turmeric in 5 Minutes

Green Side Dish of Power:

Mustard Brussels Sprouts in 5 Minutes

Week 1 (Day 6)

This day of the Healthy Weight Loss Eating Plan includes easy-to-prepare menus with exciting flavors and good nutrition; you'll have plenty of delicious foods to keep you satisfied. High-fiber cereal with fruit will be served for the High-Energy Breakfast, Chinese chicken cabbage salad with cilantro and ginger for the Power Lunch, and salmon with mustard over spinach for the Slimming Dinner. You'll also get a High-Energy Snack of orange segments, walnuts, pear, and sunflower seeds; an Appetizer Satisfier of cucumbers, bell peppers, and tomato; a Green Power Side Dish of spinach; and a Healthier Lifestyle Tea. These meals are made up of nutrient-dense foods that provide you with many of the health-promoting nutrients you require on a daily basis.

Breakfast

1 cup fiber-rich cereal

¼ cup raisins 1/4 cup strawberries

1 cup skim non-fat milk

Energizing Snack:

1 orange, medium size

four walnut halves

Lunch

Chinese Chicken Cabbage Salad with Cilantro and Ginger

Energizing Snack:

1 pear

1 tablespoon sunflower seeds

Dinner

Appetizer:

½ cup cucumber slices

½ cup red bell peppers, sliced

1 medium tomato, salmon sliced with mustard

1-Minute Spinach as a Side Dish 1

Week 1 (Day 7)

This day of the Healthy Weight Loss Eating Plan includes easy-to-prepare menus with exciting flavors and good nutrition; you'll have plenty of delicious foods to keep you satisfied. Huevos Rancheros for the High-Energy Breakfast, Lentil Salad for the Power Lunch, and Chicken Breast with Rosemary, Thyme, and Sage for the Slimming Dinner.

You'll also get a High-Energy Snack of apple, Brazil nuts, pear, and yogurt; an Appetizer Satisfier of crudite with garlic dip; a Green Power Side Dish of broccoli; and Healthier Lifestyle Tea. These meals are made up of nutrient-dense foods that provide many of the health-promoting nutrients you require on a daily basis.

Breakfast

Huevos Rancheros

½ cantaloupes, large

Snack for Energy:

1 apple, medium size

2 pistachios

Lunch

Mediterranean Lentil Salad

Energizing Snack:

1 medium-size pear

4 oz plain non-fat yogurt

Dinner

Appetizer:

Garlic Dip with 1/2 cup cucumber slices

½ cup sliced fresh red bell pepper

½ cup sliced fresh zucchini

Rosemary, Thyme, and Sage Chicken Breast Sautéed Crimini Mushrooms are a healthy option.

Week 1 of the Healthy Weight Loss Eating Plan includes 100% or more of the Daily Value for 19 health-promoting nutrients and their health benefits for long-term health. Because, as you can see, the Plan is built around nutrient-rich foods, it will help you avoid nutrient deficiencies. These foods are high in vitamins, minerals, hard-to-find omega-3 fatty acids, protein, fiber, antioxidants, and many other nutrients. The Plan's nutrient-rich foods can provide nutrients in forms that are more readily available to you than most nutritional capsules. It is also an anti-inflammatory and immunity plan because it prevents inflammation, reduces free radicals, and strengthens the immune system.

The Healthy Weight Loss Eating Plan
Week 2

Week 2 (Day 1)

This day of the Healthy Weight Loss Eating Plan includes easy-to-prepare menus with exciting flavors and good nutrition; you'll have plenty of delicious foods to keep you satisfied. Energizing Oatmeal for the High-Energy Breakfast, a Healthy Chef's Salad with Chicken, Cheddar Cheese, and Avocados for the Power Lunch, and tasty Miso Salmon with Swiss Chard for the Slimming Dinner. You'll also get a High-Energy Snack of kiwifruit, almonds, orange segments, and Brazil nuts; an Appetizer Satisfier of bell peppers, zucchini, and cucumbers; a Green Power Side Dish of Brussels sprouts; and a Healthier Lifestyle Tea. These meals are made up of nutrient-dense foods that provide you with many of the health-promoting nutrients you require on a daily basis.

Breakfast

Oatmeal

½ papaya

Snack for Energy:

2 kiwis

3 almonds

Lunch

Healthy Chef's Salad with Chicken, Cheddar Cheese, and Avocados

Energizing Snacks:

1 medium orange

1 nut of Brazil

Dinner

Appetizer:

½ cup red bell peppers, sliced

½ cup sliced zucchini

½ cup sliced cucumber

Side Dish:

Miso Salmon served with the following side dish:

Three-Minute Swiss Chard

2 Brussels Sprouts in 5 Minutes with Mustard

Week 2 (Day 2)

This day of the Healthy Weight Loss Eating Plan includes easy-to-prepare menus with exciting flavors and good nutrition; you'll have plenty of delicious foods to keep you satisfied. You'll have yogurt with fruit and sunflower seeds for the High-Energy Breakfast, a Healthy Waldorf Salad for the Power Lunch, and Healthy Sautéed Scallops for the Slimming Dinner.

You'll also get a High-Energy Snack of orange wedges, sunflower seeds, figs, and almonds, an Appetizer Satisfier of crudite with hummus, a Green Power Side Dish of broccoli and kale, and Healthier Lifestyle Tea. These meals are made up of nutrient-dense foods that provide you with many of the health-promoting nutrients you require on a daily basis.

Breakfast

8 oz nonfat plain yogurt

½ cup fresh strawberries

3 tablespoons sunflower seeds

1 medium sliced banana

Energizing Snack:

1 medium orange

1 tablespoon sunflower seeds

Lunch

Healthy Waldorf Salad

Energizing Snack:

2 dried figs

3 almonds

Dinner

Appetizer:

¼ cup bell peppers

1 cup carrot strips/slices

¼ cup sliced cucumber

Hummus from the Mediterranean

Scallops in Three Minutes

Side Dish:

Healthy Scallops sautéed in 3 minutes

Spinach in 1 Minute

3 Mediterranean Medleys in 5 Minutes

Week 2 (Day 3)

This day of the Healthy Weight Loss Eating Plan includes easy-to-prepare menus with exciting flavors and good nutrition. You'll eat plenty of delicious foods to keep you satisfied. High-fiber cereal with berries and sunflower seeds for the High-Energy Breakfast, Mexican Cheese Salad for the Power Lunch, and 7-Minute Sautéed Chicken and Asparagus for the Slimming Dinner. You'll also get a HighEnergy Snack of grapes, Brazil nuts, rye crackers, and almond butter; an Appetizer Satisfier of zucchini, bell peppers, and cucumbers; a Green Power Side Dish of collard greens; and a Healthier Lifestyle Tea. These meals are made up of nutrient-dense foods that provide you with many of the health-promoting nutrients you require on a daily basis.

Breakfast

1 cup fiber-rich cereal

¼ cup sunflower seeds 12 cup blueberries

1 cup skim nonfat milk

Energizing Snack:

1 grape cup

1 nut of Brazil

Lunch

Mexican Cheese Salad

Energizing Snack:

2 rye crisps

1 tablespoon almond butter

Dinner

Appetizer:

1 cup thinly sliced zucchini

½ cup red bell peppers, sliced

½ cup cucumber slices

Side Dish:

Green Asparagus and Sautéed Chicken in 7 Minutes 5-Minute Collard Greens arc a powerful side dish. or Broccoli

Week 2 (Day 4)

This day of the Healthy Weight Loss Eating Plan includes easy-to-prepare menus with exciting flavors and good nutrition; you'll have plenty of delicious foods to keep you satisfied. Poached Egg over Spinach and Mushrooms for the High-Energy Breakfast, Pineapple Chicken Salad for the Power Lunch, and Black Bean Chili for the Slimming Dinner.

You'll also get a High-Energy Snack of yogurt, apple, kiwifruit, and almonds, an Appetizer Satisfier of carrots, zucchini, and cucumbers, a Green Power Side Dish with spinach, and Healthier Lifestyle Tea. These meals are made up of nutrient-dense foods that provide you with many of the health-promoting nutrients you require on a daily basis.

Breakfast

Combine Healthy Sautéed Crimini Mushrooms 2 servings with 1-minute spinach and mushrooms with 2 tablespoons pumpkin seeds, 1 ounce feta cheese, and 1 poached egg, preferably a -rich egg.

1 whole wheat toast slice

Snack for Energy:

4 oz nonfat plain yogurt

½ medium apples

Lunch

Pineapple Chicken Salad

Snack for Energy:

2 kiwis

3 almonds

Dinner

Appetizer:

1 cup carrot sticks or slices

1 cup sliced zucchini

½ cup cucumber slices

Chili with Black Beans

¼ cup of brown rice

Side Dish:

1-Minute Spinach

Week 2 (Day 5)

This day of the Healthy Weight Loss Eating Plan includes easy-to-prepare menus with exciting flavors and good nutrition; you'll have plenty of delicious foods to keep you satisfied. High-Energy Breakfast Shake is served for the High-Energy Breakfast, Power Lunch Mediterranean Garbanzo Bean Salad is served for the Power Lunch, and Slimming Dinner Seared Asian Tuna is served for the Slimming Dinner. You'll also get a High-Energy Snack of apple, almonds, yogurt, and walnuts; an Appetizer Satisfier of bell peppers, zucchini, and cauliflower; a Green Power Side Dish of red cabbage (the red phytonutrients cover up the green ones); and Healthier Lifestyle Tea.

These meals are made up of nutrient-dense foods that provide you with many of the health-promoting nutrients you require on a daily basis.

Breakfast

1 apple, medium size

three almonds

Lunch

Mediterranean Garbanzo Bean Salad

Energizing Snack:

4 oz plain non-fat yogurt

1 tablespoon sunflower seeds

Dinner

Appetizer

½ cup red bell peppers, sliced

¼ cup cauliflower florets 1 cup sliced zucchini

Side Dish:

Green Seared Asian Tuna

Sautéed Red Cabbage with 2 tablespoons sunflower seeds

Sautéed Crimini Mushrooms are a healthy option.

Week 2 (Day 6)

This day of the Healthy Weight Loss Eating Plan includes easy-to-prepare menus with exciting flavors and good nutrition; you'll have plenty of delicious foods to keep you satisfied. Poached Egg over Mushrooms and Kale for the High-Energy Breakfast, Citrus Spinach Salad with Shrimp for the Power Lunch, and Halibut with Cauliflower and Fennel for the Slimming Dinner. You'll also get a High-Energy Snack of pear, almonds, yogurt, and cantaloupe; an Appetizer Satisfier of crudite with tahini; a Green Power Side Dish of collard greens; and Healthier Lifestyle Tea. These meals are made up of nutrient-dense foods that provide you with many of the health-promoting nutrients you require on a daily basis.

Breakfast

Combine Healthy Sautéed Crimini Mushrooms for a High-Energy Breakfast 1 with 5-Minute Italian Kale and 1 poached egg, preferably omega-rich.

Snack for Energy:

1 medium pear, 3 almonds

Lunch

Citrus Spinach Salad with Shrimp

Energizing Snack:

2 oz plain non-fat yogurt

½ cubed cantaloupe

Dinner

Appetizer:

½ cup carrot strips/slices

½ cup sliced cucumbers

1 cup sliced zucchini

Cauliflower and Fennel Halibut

Sautéed Shiitake Mushrooms Are Healthy

Side Dish:

Collard Greens in 5 Minutes 1 or Broccoli 1 Dessert Optional: Yogurt and Chocolate Berry Dessert in 10 Minutes

Week 2 (Day 7)

This day of the Healthy Weight Loss Eating Plan includes easy-to-prepare menus with exciting flavors and good nutrition; you'll enjoy plenty of delicious foods that will keep you satisfied. Ground Turkey with Italian Kale will be served for the High-Energy Breakfast, Tuna Salad Without Mayo for the Power Lunch, and Thai Shrimp with Basil for the Slimming Dinner.

Along with these, you'll get a High-Energy Snack of apple, almond butter, pear, and yogurt; an Appetizer Satisfier of zucchini and carrots; a Green Power Side Dish of collard greens; and Healthier Lifestyle Tea.

These meals are made up of nutrient-dense foods that provide many of the health-promoting nutrients you require on a daily basis.

Breakfast

Ground Turkey and Italian Kale

½ cantaloupe

1 slice 100% whole wheat toast

Energizing snack:

1 medium apple with 1 tablespoon almond butter

Energizing Snack:

1 medium-size pear

4 oz non-fat plain yogurt

Dinner

Appetizer:

1 cup zucchini slices

½ cup carrot slices/sticks

Side Dish:

Thai Shrimp with Basil Served with Green Power 5-Minute Collard **Optional Desserts:**

5-Minute Ginger Pineapple or 10-Minute Orange Treat

Week 2 of the Healthy Weight Loss Eating Plan includes 100% or more of the Daily Value for 19 health-promoting nutrients and their health benefits for long-term health. The Strategy will

As you can see, it is built around nutrient-rich foods that are high in vitamins, minerals, hard-to-find protein, fiber, antioxidants, and many other nutrients. The Plan's nutrient-rich foods can provide nutrients in forms that are more readily available to you than most nutritional capsules. It is also an anti-inflammatory and immunity plan because it prevents inflammation, reduces free radicals, and strengthens the immune system.

CONGRATULATIONS

Congratulations, you have now completed the first 14 days of the Plan.

When you eat the foods in the Plan, you should notice a quick response from your body. You will also feel more alert and energized as you begin to lose weight. You should repeat the two weeks you just finished to complete the 28-day weight loss plan now that this way of eating has begun to work. You'll be well on your way to a slimmer you by the end of it.

CHAPTER ELEVEN

Practical Suggestions for Maintaining Healthy Weight Loss

Tips for Eating Healthily for Weight Loss
Breakfast

Making time for a nutritious breakfast sets the tone for healthy eating throughout the day. Most people have breakfast at least 8-10 hours after their previous meal. So, in essence, you have been "fasting" while sleeping. In fact, when broken down, the word itself means "to break a fast." You may feel hungry or have low blood sugar when you wake up in the morning. Breakfast should contribute between 350 and 500 calories to your daily calorie intake.

Breakfast should provide about one-quarter of your daily protein requirements. This can be accomplished by including nuts, seeds, eggs, complex carbohydrates, and whole grain cereals in your first meal of the day.

When choosing cereal, look for one that is made from whole grains, has 5 grams of fiber per serving, and is low in sugar and salt. Avoid eating foods high in refined carbohydrates first thing in the morning (for example, sugary cereals; white flour pancakes, waffles, bagels, and muffins; or white flour-based breakfast rolls or bars).

These foods can cause a rapid spike in your blood sugar, providing you with a brief burst of energy but causing you to "crash" an hour or two later.

What happens if you skip a healthy breakfast? If you don't feed your body properly first thing in the morning, you may suffer from a variety of negative consequences, including low blood sugar levels and metabolic imbalances that leave you feeling sleepy or fatigued. And by the time lunch arrives, you'll most likely be so hungry that you'll eat anything in sight! Several studies have found that skipping breakfast increases the likelihood of becoming overweight or obese.

Many people claim that they are not hungry first thing in the morning, which makes eating breakfast difficult. Eating a smaller dinner meal will help stimulate your appetite for breakfast. If you don't have much of an appetite in the morning, start with something small, such as a half-piece of whole grain toast with nut butter or a small bowl of whole grain cereal (with no added sugars!) with milk. You may notice a greater appetite in the morning as your body adjusts to digesting food. According to recent scientific studies, those who eat breakfast every day lose more weight.

Good breakfast examples:

Green Tea with one of the following combinations:

• Energizing milk (or soy or rice milk) oatmeal with blueberries and almonds

• Whole grain breakfast cereal with fruit and nuts or seeds (sunflower or pumpkin seeds)

• Poached eggs over spinach

Tips for Eating Healthily for Weight Loss:

Lunch

The solution to the dilemma of not having enough time to prepare a healthy lunch is to prepare a salad meal for lunch. Salad meals can give you all of the nutritional benefits of the Healthiest Way to Eat without requiring you to cook!

They are quick to prepare and the varieties available are only limited by your imagination. To make a salad meal, simply put together all of the ingredients you want to include. These salad meals are not the same as the "salads" that many of us grew up with, which consisted of a bowl of iceberg lettuce topped with tomatoes and French dressing. These are nutrient-dense, nourishing meals that can be made in minutes with simple fresh ingredients.

While visiting people and cultures where there were traditionally few, if any, instances of the modern diseases that plague us today, I rediscovered the lost history of the classic Mediterranean-style salad. These were countries where people had come to expect the natural enjoyment of a long and vigorous life, such as those in the Mediterranean, including the Greek island of Crete. Salad meals were a big part of these people's diets. The Romans referred to them as salatas.

Mediterranean-style salad meals are fresh, crisp, and delicious, and they contain every nutrient imaginable. It has the potential to be one of the most enjoyable meals of the day. In fact, a salad meal made up of various types of lettuce and containing a wide variety of foods is often closer to a "complete meal" than many other food options. However, not all lettuce is the same. The darker leaf lettuces provide you with more vitamins. And the lettuce in salads contains a lot of fiber, which makes you feel full and satisfied. Furthermore, if you limit the amount of dressing used, they can be low in calories!

Here are some of the best salad greens to choose from.

• Romaine lettuce

• Spinach

• Green leaf lettuce

• Red leaf lettuce

• Boston lettuce

• Arugula

• Watercress

Topping lettuce and salad greens with chicken, seeds, nuts, fish, shellfish, or beans can provide more protein than a hamburger, twice the nutrients of a traditional "entrée" plus two "side vegetables," and hard-to-find omega-3 fatty acids. They can also have a very low glycemic index.

Even small amounts of "garnish" ingredients, such as a tablespoon of pumpkin seeds or a sprinkling of walnuts instead of croutons, are a very nutritious addition. Trace minerals and small amounts of high-quality omega-3 fats are nutrients that most Americans do not get enough of, and it doesn't take many pumpkin seeds or walnuts to incorporate some of these essential nutrients into the day's Healthiest Way of Eating.

Consider a salad meal to be a blank canvas on which to mix various "colors" of foods. You can make a salad with a mixture of your favorite lettuces depending on your mood, the season, and the contents of your refrigerator. Starting with a nutrient-dense lettuce like romaine and incorporating a mesclun or spring mix variety of lettuces will provide a solid foundation for any salad. You can then add a variety of leafy greens, root vegetables, or other vegetables.

The possibilities for nutrient-rich food combinations are endless. You can then add fruit, nuts, seeds, beans, legumes, and so on. The list of things you can add to a salad meal to make it more delicious and nutritious is endless. Combine a variety of foods that contain a wide range of nutrients, and your salad bowl may one day replace your multivitamin supplement.

And don't forget the dressing. The fats in dressings are required for our bodies to absorb carotenoids—the red, yellow, and orange pigments found in fruits and vegetables that act as antioxidants and prevent free radical damage that promotes aging and chronic disease. This is because carotenoids (along with vitamins A, D, and E) are fat-soluble, which means they cannot be absorbed unless there is fat present. According to research, adding a little fat to your salads can significantly increase the amount of protective compounds you absorb. People who use full-fat dressing absorb twice as many nutrients as those who use reduced-fat dressing. And there was no absorption among those who used nonfat dressing!

Eating a salad meal is one of the simplest and healthiest eating habits you can adopt. You can have a health-promoting meal with enough protein, healthy fats, vitamins, minerals, and powerful antioxidants to last you the entire afternoon in just 5 minutes.

Tips for Eating Healthily for Weight Loss

Dinner

There are three basic don'ts when it comes to dinner and how it may affect your sleep, according to nutritional research. First, don't make your dinner meal too large, especially in terms of food volume and fat content. Large amounts of food simply take too long for your stomach to empty. According to some studies, about 10-15 grams of fat in food can be processed in the stomach and passed on to the small intestine in one hour. It's not uncommon for one fried chicken breast to contain 20 grams of fat and one large serving of French fries to contain 30 grams of fat. The 50 grams of fat in those two foods may increase digestion time in the stomach to 5 hours! If you ate these two foods at 8:00 p.m., it could be 1:00 a.m. before they left your stomach. (During the night, excessive gastric acid secretion in your stomach can be a factor that disrupts sleep.) As a general rule, you should keep your dinners between 350 and 550 calories, and your dinner fats should be no more than 10-15 grams. That usually means no fried foods and only a few tablespoons of fat-laden sauces and salad dressings.

The second don't has to do with the glycemic index. Although I've seen some research and Internet discussion about high-glycemic index foods and their benefits for sleep, I believe that the best research and the healthiest approach here is to stick with low-GI foods at dinner (and at other meals as well). Several studies have shown that eating low-GI foods at dinner can improve blood sugar reactions after breakfast the next morning and help the rest of the day start out better for your blood sugar balance.

Breakfast and lunch should provide you with the nourishment and energy you need to get through the rest of the day. When you eat dinner (unless you work a late shift or have responsibilities that require you to deviate from the natural cycle of waking hours in the daylight and sleeping hours in the dark), you are no longer preparing for the activities of the day.

Instead, you're attempting to get a good night's sleep so that you can wake up refreshed the next day. Low-GI foods, in my opinion, are the best way to help you achieve this goal. Green leafy vegetables, cruciferous vegetables, and salad-type vegetables (such as lettuce, tomatoes, celery, bell peppers, radish, and cucumbers) have the lowest GI values of any food group and can be particularly beneficial here. Processed and refined grain products (such as breads and pastas that are not made from 100% whole grains) and sugar-added foods or drinks are on the no-no list.

The third and final point does not involve timing. You don't want to eat your dinner too soon before going to bed. Your digestive tract works best when you are upright, and sleeping does not allow your stomach to work overtime. If you keep your dinner meals in the 350-550 calorie and 10-15 grams of fat range that I recommend, you should be able to eat your dinner meal 3-4 hours before bedtime and have it work with your sleep.

As previously stated, low-GI and moderate-fat foods are good options for dinner. In the low-GI category, you should focus on the following vegetables: green leafy vegetables, cruciferous vegetables, and salad-type vegetables such as lettuce, tomatoes, celery, bell peppers, radishes, and cucumbers.

If you're going to include starchy vegetables like potatoes or green peas, I recommend keeping the serving size to _-1 cup. Whole grains are also good options here, but keep them to 1 cup or less.

Protein-containing foods are another "do" for dinner.

Some research studies have shown that combining low-GI carbs and protein at dinner can help improve sleep, and there is some evidence that one specific amino acid—tryptophan—has a better chance of playing a helpful role in our sleep-related nervous system activity when we combine dinner foods that provide protein and low-GI carbs. Fish is an excellent source of protein in this situation (but stay away from fried or breaded fish). If you enjoy and perform well on lean meats, they can also be a good source of protein and should be kept in the 4-6 ounce range at dinner.

The importance of a relaxed, enjoyable meal is a final "do" when it comes to dinner meals! Because dinner is so close to bedtime, it's especially important to chew thoroughly and relax in a way that allows your body to engage in optimal digestion. At dinnertime, stick with some healthy protein choices (like non-fried fish) and low-GI (glycemic index) foods (like fresh green vegetables) to enjoy the smells, textures, and flavors of the World's Healthiest Foods. As a general rule, keep your dinner meal between 350-550 calories and 10-15 grams of fat. Don't overdo it on any food, and leave at least 3-4 hours between dinner and bedtime. Also, treat your dinner as the type of meal that is intended to be especially relaxing and enjoyable.

Tips for Eating Healthily for Weight Loss

Snacks

Healthy snacks contain an adequate amount of protein, fats, fiber, and accompanying nutrients that not only satiate your appetite so you are less hungry between meals, but also provide you with health-promoting nutrients to provide you with long-lasting energy.

Snacks should also provide energy and a sense of fullness while consuming the fewest calories. That's why I don't recommend popular snacks like energy bars because they contain excess fats and sweeteners, which add empty calories to your daily calorie quota. While a small amount of fat helps to maintain satiety, too much fat can slow down digestion to the point where it takes too long to get energy and nourishment from your food. Furthermore, excessive amounts of simple sugars can cause you to become hungry very quickly—much before your next meal. They also lack fresh ingredients, which can help boost your energy and vitality.

Fresh fruit (such as apples, pears, and blueberries) combined with nuts (such as almonds, walnuts, and cashews) is an example of a healthy snack because it provides a good combination of fiber from the fruit and protein from the nuts (the latter increases the snack's "holding power"). The fats in the almonds help to slow the digestive process and extend the snack's impact. Fresh fruit and yogurt make an excellent healthy snack combination. These snacks are not only healthy, but they are also less expensive than pre-packaged energy bars.

I'd like to add one more set of observations about people who snack excessively. It's critical to consider the overall pattern of your day in terms of enjoyment and activities. You may or may not want to make healthy snacking the solution to a daily pattern that isn't bringing you balance and enjoyment. In some cases, planning a larger, more nourishing meal before a difficult snack period—and then shifting activities to turn a former snack period into a period of time focused on other enjoyable pursuits—can be a more effective way of "tiding yourself over" than experimenting with snack content.

Tips for Eating Healthily for Weight Loss

Appetizer

Even when I cook for myself, I make appetizers like broccoli and cauliflower florets, cucumbers, red bell peppers, and zucchini and serve them with a healthy dip like guacamole or hummus. These are some of the healthiest and simplest appetizers to make. Extra virgin olive oil, balsamic vinegar, low-fat yogurt, and nut/seed butters, such as almond butter or tahini (sesame seed butter), also make excellent no-prep dips. These are more appealing to me than the more traditional soup and salad appetizers, and they can be healthier and easier to prepare.

Even though it is not difficult to cut and chop the vegetables yourself, you may want to consider the added convenience of pre-chopped and pre-sliced vegetables (though they are slightly more expensive). Many stores sell organically grown, pre-cut vegetables, which may provide just the right amount of extra convenience to get you started on some new appetizer ideas.

It is frequently recommended to soak vegetables in ice water for one hour before serving. I would avoid this method because soaking removes many (about 20) of the nutrients found in vegetables.

Appetizers made up of vegetable-plus-dip combinations will satisfy your hunger while also preventing overeating once the meal is served. Healthy appetizers are usually around 100 calories.

My picks for the best healthy appetizers include fresh vegetable crudités served with accompaniments like:

- Hummus

- Guacamole

- Tahini

- Salsa

- Olive tapenade

- Nut butters

Tips for Eating Healthily for Weight Loss

Beverages

Most people understand, to varying degrees, that what they eat (or don't eat) affects their overall health. As a result of this recognition, many people try to eat more fruits and vegetables, less saturated fat and cholesterol, and avoid junk foods.

It is important to remember, however, that what you drink (or do not drink) has an impact on your health. If you eat well but consume excessive amounts of soda, fruit juice, coffee, and/or alcoholic beverages, you may not be as healthy as you could be. This is because such beverages contain a variety of substances that, when consumed in excess, are harmful to one's health. Refined or artificial sweeteners, artificial flavorings, artificial colorings, synthetic preservatives, caffeine, and alcohol are examples of these substances. Here are my recommendations for keeping your beverage choices at the same peak nourishment level as your food choices:

Water: You can't go wrong with good water. This beverage is not only at the top of my list, but it is in a class by itself. While your water intake needs will vary from day to day, the National Academy of Sciences recommends 13 cups of water per day for men and 9 cups for women in its Dietary Reference Intake (DRI) recommendations. Space your intake throughout the day, rehydrate before and after exercise, and avoid excessive water consumption during meal times if you find that practice beneficial. I recommend attaching a high-quality filter to your tap water supply and drinking this filtered tap water as your primary source of water for the best water. To ensure that you have easy access to home-filtered water, buy an easy-to-carry water bottle and refill it whenever you are at home so that you can have water with you when you are on the go. Look for ones made of glass or stainless steel. If you're getting a hard plastic (polycarbonate) bottle, be sure to purchase a "BPA-free" one.

(BPA is an abbreviation for bisphenol A, a toxic toxin that is frequently added to polycarbonate plastics.)

100% pure fruit juices: Fruit juice can be healthy if it is made entirely of fruit juice and contains no added sweeteners. However, keep in mind that juice can pack a powerful punch in terms of calories and sugar, so if you are trying to lose weight or have blood sugar regulation concerns, it may not be wise to consume a lot of juice, even 100% fruit juice. To get the most out of the nutrients in the fruit, press or juice it at home and consume it right away. If you want to buy fruit juice at the grocery store, keep in mind that it is more difficult to find 100% fruit juice than you might think because many fruit beverages sold in supermarkets contain only a small percentage (usually less than 10%) of actual fruit juice. Instead of soda, make a refreshing and healthy punch for a special occasion by combining sparkling water, 100%

cranberry juice, ice, and orange slices in a large bowl. (Remember, though, that while 100% fruit juice is a healthy beverage, it should not be mistaken for whole fresh fruit.)

Herbal iced tea:

Instead of regular iced tea, try a refreshing glass of herbal iced tea. Many herbs contain high levels of antioxidants, which help the immune system and overall health. Brew the tea stronger than you would if serving it hot, and then add ice and a sprig of mint or a slice of lemon. When served cold, peppermint tea is delicious. Alternatively, combine chamomile, hibiscus flower, lemon grass, orange peel, rose hips, and strawberry leaf.

Tea for a Healthier Lifestyle:

Healthier Lifestyle Tea is the name I've given to a tasty and healthy beverage made with one cup of green tea and one teaspoon of lemon juice. Green tea is not only tasty, but it is also known for its health-promoting properties.

These have been linked to its high concentration of catechin phytonutrients, which have a wide range of protective benefits, many of which are associated with their powerful ability to fight free radicals. Adding 1 teaspoon of lemon juice to each cup of green tea not only adds a refreshing flavor but also provides additional benefits. Lemon juice is a concentrated source of vitamin C, and a hot water and lemon beverage is both cleansing and energizing. If you are caffeine sensitive, you can drink decaffeinated green tea. Green tea is best enjoyed hot without sweeteners; however, stevia, agave nectar, or honey are the best options for sweetening your green tea.

Red Wine:

Red wine has been linked to a variety of health benefits. Always drink wine with your meals. The current recommendations are one glass per day for women and two glasses per day for men. If you cannot tolerate alcohol or prefer not to include it in your diet, you can reap the benefits of resveratrol by drinking alcohol-free red wine or purple grape juice.

CHAPTER TWELVE

The Healthiest Cooking Method

Cooking has been a passion of mine since I was five years old.

I attended some of the world's best culinary schools, including La Varenne in Paris, Guiliano Bugialli's cooking school in Florence, and Gourmet's Oxford in England. My cooking and food development experience (when I ran Health Valley Foods) inspired me to develop recipes and food preparation techniques that enhanced the health benefits of foods. This is the healthiest way to cook, in my opinion.

In addition to selecting the World's Healthiest Foods as the foundation of your Healthiest Way of Eating, it is critical to prepare them in ways that preserve their nutrient-richness. That's because the nutritional quality of a food (say, a vegetable) that has been cooked enough to have enhanced taste and texture versus one that has been overcooked is vastly different.

To reap the full benefits of the World's Healthiest Foods, cook them for the shortest amount of time possible in order to preserve their health-promoting compounds. That's why, in my book, The World's Healthiest Foods: Essential Guide for the Healthiest Way of Eating (and those I featured in the Healthy Weight Loss Eating Plan), most of the Healthiest Way of Cooking recommendations for vegetables (and those I featured in the Healthy Weight Loss Eating Plan) take only five minutes or less. You can cook vegetables al dente—tender on the outside, crisp on the inside—in this short amount of time, giving them a delightful texture and vibrant flavor while retaining far more nutrients than if you cooked them for longer. Following my recommendations for the best cooking method and cooking time for each of the World's Healthiest Foods, as outlined in The World's Healthiest Foods book and the recipes included in this e-book, will ensure you enjoy delicious foods that are also nutritious.

In addition to preserving nutrients during cooking, it is critical to cook foods in ways that do not produce harmful compounds. Cooking with oil, for example, can oxidize the fats and produce lipid peroxidation products, which can cause problems in the body and increase the risk of atherosclerosis. Instead of using oil, I developed a healthy cooking method called Healthy Sauté, which uses vegetable or chicken broth.

Healthy Sauté is a unique method of food preparation because it combines three methods into one. It's a sauté that uses vegetable or chicken broth instead of heated oils; I'm especially conscious of creating recipes that don't use heated oils because they can be harmful to your health. It is similar to stir-frying in that it brings out the robust flavor of foods while cooking them at a lower temperature. It's similar to steaming in that there's enough moisture to soften the cellulose and hemicellulose, which improves digestibility. A small amount of liquid is required for Healthy Sauté to keep the vegetables moist and tender. Because steaming and boiling dilute the flavor of vegetables like cauliflower and asparagus, which only require a small amount of liquid to tenderize, they are excellent candidates for Healthy Sauté.

Step-by-Step Healthy Sauté

• In a stainless steel skillet, heat 3-5 tablespoons broth.

• When the broth begins to steam, add the vegetables, cover if necessary, and sauté for the recommended amount of time.

Aside from reducing your exposure to oxidized oils, another great benefit of Healthy Sauté that is inherently important to healthy weight loss is the reduction of calorie consumption. Consider this... When sautéing vegetables, a few tablespoons of oil is typically used. All you really get from the oil is the texture, and you don't always get much flavor. However, two tablespoons of oil can add over 200 calories to your meal. You can save the majority of these calories by sautéing with broth rather than oil. You probably agree that that's a lot of calories that could be used better.

One more thing about oil: as you can see, extra virgin olive oil is an important component of the Mediterranean diet, and it is also one of the foods (and the only oil) listed as a World's Healthiest Food. However, I do not recommend cooking with it because the monounsaturated fats and polyphenol antioxidants in it can be damaged. Instead, I recommend incorporating it into salads and dressings, as well as drizzling it over vegetables, fish, and chicken. (I believe the highest heat it can withstand is when making sauces.)

How to Get the Most Out of Alllium and Cruciferous Vegetables

If you let your allium or cruciferous vegetables sit for 5-10 minutes after cutting them, you can help boost their health-promoting properties.

Allium vegetables

According to the most recent scientific research, slicing, chopping, mincing, or pressing allium vegetables (such as garlic, onions, and leeks) before cooking increases the health-promoting properties of garlic. When garlic is whole, its cell structure separates a sulphur-based compound called alliin and an enzyme called alliinase. Cutting garlic ruptures the cells and releases these elements allowing them to come in contact and form a powerful new compound called alliin which not only adds to the number of garlic's health-promoting benefits but is also the culprit behind their pungent aroma and gives garlic its "bite".

When it comes to garlic, the finer the cut, the more alliin is produced. The strongest flavor and the most alliin are obtained by pressing or mincing garlic into a smooth paste. The stronger the smell and flavor of garlic, the more nutrients it contains. So, the next time you chop, mince, or press garlic, you may appreciate its strong aroma even more, knowing that the more pungent the smell, the better it is for your health!

Because this is a time-consuming process, I recommend letting the garlic sit for 5-10 minutes after cutting while you prepare the other ingredients. This is done to maximize alliin synthesis. Once formed, the compounds are quite stable and can withstand low heat for a short period of time, about 15 minutes. Garlic research supports the efficacy of this practice. The ability of crushed garlic to inhibit cancer development in animals was inhibited when heated; however, when the researchers allowed the crushed garlic to "stand" for 10 minutes before heating, its anticancer activity was preserved.

Cutting cruciferous vegetables (i.e., cabbage, kale, broccoli, cauliflower, mustard greens, etc.) into small pieces also breaks down cell walls and increases the activation of an enzyme called myrosinase, which slowly converts some of the plant nutrients into their active forms, which have been shown to have health-promoting properties. To reap the full benefits of these vegetables, allow them to sit for at least 5 minutes, preferably 10 minutes, after cutting before eating or cooking.

Heat will inactivate the effect of myrosinase, so allow the cruciferous vegetables to sit for 5-10 minutes before cooking to allow the enzyme ample time to increase the concentration of active phytonutrients. Cooking at low or medium heat for short periods of time (up to 15 minutes) should not destroy the active phytonutrients because they are fairly stable once formed.

Because ascorbic acid (vitamin C) stimulates myrosinase activity, you can sprinkle a little lemon juice on the cruciferous vegetable before cooking to boost its beneficial phytonutrient concentration even more.

CHAPTER THIRTEEN

Breakfast and Snack Recipes

Energizing Oatmeal

A fantastic way to start the day! And who would have guessed that a bowl of oatmeal could provide your Healthy Weight Loss Plan with so many nutrients?

Ingredients:

2 cups of water

1 cup rolled oats, old fashioned

¼ cup raisins 1 apple, chopped

¼ cup cranberries, dried

½ teaspoon cinnamon

1 tablespoon ground flax seeds

1 tablespoon chopped walnuts

1 cup skim milk

1 tablespoon blackstrap molasses

Directions:

1. In a saucepan, bring the water and salt to a boil, then reduce to a low heat and add the oats, chopped apple, raisins, and dried cranberries.

2. Cook for about 5 minutes, stirring frequently to prevent the oatmeal from clumping together. Stir in the cinnamon, flax seeds, and walnuts before covering the pan and turning off the heat. Allow for a 5-minute rest. Serve with milk and molasses on the side.

Ground turkey with kale from Italy

Breakfast with Italian kale is a great way to add nutrition to your Healthy Weight Loss menu.

Ingredients:

2 cloves garlic

½ medium onion

2 tablespoons low-sodium chicken or vegetable broth

¼ pound low-fat ground turkey

6 cups Italian kale

Season with salt and pepper to taste

Directions:

1. Chop the garlic and onion and set aside for at least 5 minutes to bring out their beneficial properties.

1. Heat 2 tablespoons broth over medium heat. Sauté the onion for 3 minutes, stirring frequently.

2. Add the garlic and turkey and cook for 3 minutes more, breaking up the clumps of turkey.

3. Cook for 5 minutes the kale.

4. Combine the steamed kale with the turkey mixture. Season to taste with salt and pepper.

Tea for a Healthier Lifestyle

A Healthier Way of Life Green tea with lemon is tea. It's a refreshing and energizing way to begin the day. If you are caffeine sensitive, you can drink decaffeinated green tea.

Green tea is not only tasty, but it is also known for its health-promoting properties. These have been linked to its high concentration of catechin phytonutrients, which have a wide range of protective benefits, many of which are associated with their powerful ability to fight free radicals. Adding 1 teaspoon lemon juice to each cup of green tea not only adds a refreshing flavor but also provides additional benefits. Lemon juice is a concentrated source of vitamin C, and a hot water and lemon beverage is both cleansing and energizing.

Ingredients:

a cup of green tea

1 teaspoon lemon juice

Directions:

1. Bring a non-reactive pot or pan (glass or stainless steel) to a temperature of 160-170F.

2. Pour 1 cup hot water over 1 teaspoon green tea in a sieve or tea ball.

3. After 2-3 minutes, add the lemon juice. If you steep it for too long, it will become bitter.

Green tea is not only tasty, but it is also known for its health-promoting properties. These have been linked to its high concentration of catechin phytonutrients, which have a wide range of protective benefits, many of which are associated with their powerful ability to fight free radicals. Adding 1 teaspoon lemon juice to each cup of green tea not only adds a refreshing flavor but also provides additional benefits. Lemon juice contains a high concentration of vitamin C, and a hot water and lemon drink is both cleansing and energizing.

Breakfast Shake

Quick, simple, and healthy—a great way to start the day on the go and low in calories.

Ingredients:

1 banana, medium

½ cup fresh strawberries

2 cup non-fat milk

1 tablespoon almond butter

2 tablespoons ground flaxseeds

1 tablespoon blackstrap molasses

2 tablespoons sunflower seeds

Directions:

Grind the sunflower seeds, then add the remaining ingredients and blend until smooth.

Papaya with Lime (or grapefruit in place of papaya)

Papayas are high in vitamin C, potassium, and folate and low in calories, making them an excellent addition to our Healthy Weight Loss Plan.

Ingredients:

12 grapefruit (or 1 medium papaya)

1 tablespoon lime juice

¼ teaspoon lime zest

Directions:

Cut the papaya in half and serve with the lime juice and zest.

Poached Huevos Rancheros

This simple version of a popular Mexican dish will add flavor and nutrition to your weight loss menu.

Ingredients:

3 tbsp chicken or vegetable broth (low sodium)

2 cups black beans, cooked (or 1 15 oz can of black beans, drained)

1 teaspoon cumin

¾ teaspoon red chili powder

2 tbsp fresh cilantro, chopped

Season with salt and black pepper to taste.

2 cups romaine lettuce, shredded

½ cubed large avocado

1-½ cup prepared salsa

2 poached eggs (preferably omega-rich eggs)

Directions:

1. Heat broth, beans, cumin, and red chili powder over medium low heat for about 10 minutes, stirring occasionally. Add the cilantro, salt, and pepper to taste.

2. Arrange the beans on a plate with a poached egg, salsa, shredded romaine lettuce, and avocado.

Tropical Energy Smoothie

With this quick-and-easy smoothie, you can add a touch of the tropics to your Weight Loss Plan; the tahini adds protein to help you get through the morning. It's also low in calories!

Ingredients:

2 tablespoons tahini

1 banana, medium ripe

1 cup plain non-fat yogurt

1 to ½ cup pineapple juice

1 large papaya

Directions:

Scoop out the flesh of the papaya with a spoon and add it to the blender with the rest of the ingredients. Blend until completely smooth.

Lunch and Salad Recipes

Salad with Chinese Chicken and Cabbage

Chinese cabbage, like other members of the cabbage family, is low in calories while providing the highest concentration of B vitamins, folate, and zinc.

Ingredients:

8 cups thinly sliced Napa cabbage

1 teaspoon tamari (soy sauce)

1 tablespoon minced ginger

2 medium garlic cloves, pressed

½ cup cilantro, chopped

4 oz cooked chicken breast, shredded or cut into 1-inch cubes

½ medium sliced avocado

2 tablespoons extra virgin olive oil

2 tablespoons rice vinegar

Directions:

Season with salt and pepper to taste.

Toss all salad ingredients with olive oil and vinegar before serving.

Citrus Spinach with Shrimp Salad

Baby spinach is a popular salad ingredient. Enjoy this low-calorie, nutritious salad; the oranges provide plenty of vitamin C!

Ingredients:

12 cup baby spinach, fresh

2 medium oranges, cut into small segments

2 tablespoons chopped dates

4 ounces cooked shrimp

2 tablespoons lemon juice

2 tablespoons extra virgin olive oil

Season with salt and pepper to taste.

Directions:

Toss salad ingredients with lemon juice and extra virgin olive oil.

Greece Salad with Garbanzo Beans and Feta Cheese

Salads with garbanzo beans are popular throughout the Mediterranean.

This version is not only nutritious and flavorful, but the addition of mint makes it wonderfully refreshing.

Ingredients:

12 cup salad (mixed greens)

½ cup peppermint leaves

2 oz. low-fat feta cheese

1 to ½ cup garbanzo beans

2 tablespoons sunflower seeds

½ medium avocado

Season with salt and pepper to taste.

2 tablespoons extra virgin olive oil

2 tablespoons red wine vinegar

Directions:

Toss the salad ingredients with the olive oil and vinegar.

Salad with Cheddar Cheese and Garbanzo Beans

Variety is essential for enjoying and sticking to your Healthy Weight Loss menu. This salad is a great example of how creative you can be in creating a delicious low-calorie salad.

Ingredients:

8 cups salad (mixed greens)

½ cup sliced cucumber, unpeeled 2 oz low-fat cheddar cheese, shredded

½ cup ripe red tomato

½ cup chopped fresh sweet red bell peppers 1 cup diced avocado

2 garbanzo bean cups

1 cup sliced crimini mushrooms 12 cup raisins

2 tablespoons sunflower seeds

2 tablespoons extra virgin olive oil

1 tablespoon balsamic vinegar/lemon juice

Season with salt and pepper to taste.

Directions:

Toss all salad ingredients with olive oil, vinegar, and lemon juice.

Chef Salad with Chicken, Cheddar Cheese, and Avocados

Salads are delicious, but they are only limited by your imagination. The protein from the chicken and cheddar cheese will keep you full until your mid-day snack.

Ingredients:

12 cup salad (mixed greens)

2 oz shredded or cubed chicken breast

½ cup sliced cucumbers 1 oz low-fat cheddar cheese

½ cup tomatoes, diced

½ cup red bell peppers

½ cup fresh crimini mushrooms,

½ medium avocado,

½ cup frozen green peas,

thawed garbanzo beans, ½ cup

1 tablespoon of extra virgin olive oil

1 tablespoon lemon juice

Season with salt and pepper to taste.

Directions:

Toss all salad ingredients with olive oil and lemon juice before serving.

Salad Waldorf Style

This low-calorie version of the classic Waldorf salad not only fills you up, but it's also simple to make and delicious!

Ingredients:

1 medium chopped apple

1 celery stalk, diced 4 oz-wt chicken breast, diced

2 tablespoons chopped walnuts

2 tablespoons sunflower seeds

1/2 tablespoons extra virgin olive oil 2 tablespoons chopped parsley

2 tablespoons lemon juice

12 cups mixed salad greens

Season with salt and pepper to taste.

Directions:

Combine all ingredients except the salad greens and serve over the salad greens.

Mediterranean Caesar Salad

One of the advantages of the Mediterranean diet is the abundance of vegetables and legumes, which are high in dietary fiber and help you feel satiated and satisfied—an important factor in any Healthy Weight Loss Plan.

Ingredients:

12 romaine lettuce cups

2 medium sliced or diced red tomatoes

1/2 cup sliced cucumbers, peeled

1-pound kidney beans (or legume of your choice)

1 cup crimini mushrooms, sliced

2 tablespoons grated Parmesan cheese

Dressing:

4 tablespoons lemon juice

1 tablespoon of extra virgin olive oil

2 chopped garlic cloves (optional)

Season with salt and pepper to taste.

Directions:

Toss all ingredients together with the dressing ingredients. Before tossing, the dressing ingredients do not need to be combined separately.

Mediterranean Garbanzo Beans Salad

Garbanzo beans, for example, provide a great combination of protein and fiber, both of which help you feel satisfied until your next meal.

Ingredients:

12 cup green salad

1 cup garbanzo beans

4 tablespoons chopped red onion

2 tablespoons Parmesan cheese

2 chopped medium tomatoes

2 tablespoons extra virgin olive oil

2 tablespoons lemon juice

Season with salt and pepper to taste.

Directions:

Toss all salad ingredients with olive oil and lemon juice.

Mediterranean Lentils Salad

Lentils, unlike beans, do not need to be soaked before cooking and can be prepared in 20-30 minutes. They are an excellent source of molybdenum and folate in your Healthy Weight Loss Plan.

Ingredients:

2 cups lentils, cooked

1/2 medium red onion

diced 2 garlic cloves

diced 1/2 cup tomatoes

diced 1/2 cup red bell pepper

2 teaspoons fresh lemon juice

1 tablespoon of extra virgin olive oil

4 tablespoons sunflower seeds

4 romaine lettuce cups

Season with salt and pepper to taste.

Directions:

1. Chop the garlic and set it aside for 5 minutes to release its health-promoting properties.

2. Toss together all of the ingredients. Serve alongside romaine lettuce.

Mediterranean Turkey Salad with Mushrooms

If you want to increase your intake of selenium, B vitamins, and copper, you might be surprised to learn that crimini mushrooms are an excellent source of these essential nutrients.

Ingredients:

12 cup green salad

1 medium diced tomato

1 cup cucumber slices

8 olives kalamata

2 ounces turkey breast

1 cup sliced crimini mushrooms

Dressing:

2 tablespoons extra virgin olive oil

1 tablespoon lemon juice

1 garlic clove, chopped (optional)

Season with salt and pepper to taste.

Directions:

Toss all of the ingredients together with the dressing. Before tossing, the dressing ingredients do not need to be combined separately.

Mexican Cheese Salad

Enjoy the health-promoting anthocyanins found in black beans, which not only give them their beautiful dark color but also provide you with protection against free radical activity, in this simple addition to your Healthy Weight Loss Plan.

Ingredients:

8 cups salad mix

2 cups black or pinto beans, cooked (or 1 15-oz can, rinsed and drained)

1/2 medium avocado

1 medium tomato, diced

2 oz. whole milk cheddar cheese, grated

1/4 cup salsa

To taste, lime wedge juice

Season with salt and pepper to taste.

Directions:

1. Divide the greens between two plates. Toss greens with beans, avocado, and tomato.

2. Garnish with cheddar cheese, your favorite salsa, and lime wedges.

Pineapple Chicken Salad

This unusual combination of ingredients not only tastes delicious, but the low-calorie pineapple adds an extra boost of vitamin C for antioxidant protection and immune support.

Ingredients:

2 cup pineapple, diced

2 fennel bulbs, thinly sliced

1/2 cup chicken breast, diced

3 tablespoons extra virgin olive oil

1 tablespoon lemon juice

12 cup green salad

Season with salt and pepper to taste.

Directions:

Except for the salad greens, combine all of the ingredients. Top salad greens with half of the Pineapple Chicken Salad mixture and serve.

Romaine Salad with Goat Cheese and Mushrooms

Adding salmon or sardines to a Healthy Weight Loss Salad is an easy way to help meet the recommended intake of those hard-to-find omega-3 fatty acids that are so important for optimal health.

Ingredients:

2 oz-wt sardines or canned salmon

12 cups chopped fresh romaine lettuce

1 cup sliced fresh crimini mushrooms

12 cup frozen green peas, thawed 2 medium tomatoes, diced 3 oz low-fat soft goat cheese

2 tbsp sunflower seeds

Dressing:

1 tablespoon extra virgin olive oil

2 fresh garlic cloves

2 tsp fresh lemon juice

Season with salt and pepper to taste

Directions:

Toss all ingredients with dressing. Dressing ingredients do not need to be combined separately before tossing.

Tuna Salad Without Mayo

If you didn't think you could eat tuna salad without mayo, try this unique version that is low in calories while still tasting delicious.

Ingredients:

1/2 6 oz can light tuna packed in water

2 chopped garlic cloves

1 tablespoon Dijon mustard

1 teaspoon honey

4 teaspoons fresh lemon juice

2 oz. weight soft silken tofu

1/2 cup chopped celery 8 sliced olives

2 tablespoons sunflower seeds

1 medium diced avocado

8 cups salad mix

Season with salt and pepper to taste.

Directions:

1. Chop the garlic and set it aside for 5 minutes to release its health-promoting properties.

2. Combine all ingredients except the avocado and salad greens in a mixing bowl.

3. On a plate, layer 4 cups of greens and half of the avocado, then top with half of the Tuna Without Mayo recipe.

3-Minute Scallops

Healthy Sauté your scallops for a delicious dish without the use of heated oils, which are not only unhealthy but also add extra calories when trying to lose weight.

Ingredients:

1/3-pound bay or sea scallops

1 tablespoon low-sodium chicken or vegetable broth 2 medium garlic cloves, chopped

1 tablespoon of extra virgin olive oil

1 tablespoon fresh lemon juice

Season with salt and pepper to taste.

Directions:

1. Chop garlic and set aside for 5 minutes to maximize its health-promoting properties.

2. Bring 2 quarts of water to a boil over high heat.

3. In a stainless-steel skillet, heat 1 tablespoon broth over medium heat.

4. When the broth starts to steam, add the scallops and garlic and cook for 2 minutes, stirring constantly. After 2 minutes, flip the scallops and cook for 1 minute on the

other side. Scallops cook quickly, so keep an eye on the cooking time. Scallops that have been overcooked become tough. (If you're using larger sea scallops, cook them for 1-2 minutes longer.)

5. Toss with olive oil, lemon juice, garlic, salt, and pepper.

7-Minute Sauté ed Chicken and Asparagus

When you make this delicious chicken and asparagus Healthy Weight Loss meal, you'll be getting a lot of protein and folate.

Ingredients:

2 medium garlic cloves, pressed

3 tablespoons chicken broth

½ pound boneless, skinless chicken breasts, cut into 1-inch cubes

1 to ½ pound asparagus, cut into 1-inch pieces (about 2 cups when cut)

2 teaspoon lemon juice

1 tsp red chili flakes

1/2 tablespoons extra virgin olive oil

Season with salt and white pepper to taste.

Directions:

1. Chop garlic and set aside for at least 5 minutes to extract its health benefits.

2. In a stainless-steel wok or 12-inch skillet, heat 3 tablespoons broth. Cook for 3-4 minutes after the broth begins to steam.

3. Stir in the asparagus, lemon juice, and red pepper flakes. Cover and stir together. Cook for an additional 2-3 minutes. If the asparagus is thick, cook for an additional couple of minutes. Mix in the extra virgin olive oil. Season to taste with salt and pepper.

Black Bean Chili

A filling, hearty, and flavorful vegetarian Weight Loss meal that only takes about 30 minutes to prepare.

Ingredients:

1 medium chopped onion

2 garlic cloves, minced or pressed

2 cups black beans, cooked (1 15 oz can black beans, rinsed)

1 can (15 oz) diced tomatoes

2 tablespoons chili powder

½ cup fresh cilantro

Directions:

1. Chop onions and mince or press garlic; set aside for at least 5 minutes to allow their health-promoting properties to develop.

2. Combine all ingredients (except cilantro) in a pot, cover, and simmer for 20 minutes.

3. Garnish with cilantro before serving.

Chicken Breast with Rosemary, Thyme and Sage

Herbs and spices are a low-calorie way to season almost any Healthy Weight Loss dish.

Ingredients:

2 garlic cloves, chopped

2 oz. wt chicken breast, cut into cubes

1 tablespoon fresh lemon juice

4 cup low-fat organic chicken or vegetable broth

2 teaspoons fresh sage

2 teaspoons fresh thyme

2 teaspoons fresh rosemary

Season with salt and pepper to taste.

Directions:

1. Chop garlic and set aside for 5 minutes to bring out its health benefits.

2. Cut the chicken into pieces and season with lemon juice, salt, and pepper.

3. Heat the broth, then add the chicken and herbs. Cook for 3-4 minutes, or until the chicken is thoroughly cooked.

Halibut with Ginger and Scallions

Include this tasty low-calorie Asian-flavored dish on your Healthy Weight Loss menu. It's one of our favorites because it's high in protein and low in fat.

Ingredients:

¼-pound halibut, cut into two pieces

2 tbsp chicken or vegetable broth (low sodium)

1 tablespoon mirin rice wine* 1 medium garlic clove, chopped

½ teaspoon tamari (soy sauce) 12 teaspoon fresh lemon juice

½ teaspoon minced fresh ginger

½ cup scallions, coarsely chopped

* Japanese rice cooking wine, found in the Asian section of the market, to taste

Directions:

1. Chop garlic and set aside for 5 minutes to allow its health-promoting properties to develop.

2. Heat the broth in a 10-inch skillet over medium-high heat.

3. Combine the garlic, tamari, lemon juice, ginger, and scallions in a mixing bowl.

4. Arrange halibut steaks on top, cover, and reduce heat to low. Cook for 5 minutes, depending on the thickness. Season with salt and pepper to taste.

Remove the steaks and place them on a plate. Serve the fish with the ginger and scallion mixture.

Mediterranean Cod with Red Bell Peppers and Basil

Healthy weight loss is all about combining great taste, great nutrition, and a low calories count. This recipe succeeds on all three counts.

Ingredients:

¼ pound cod fillets

2 tablespoons plus ½ cup low-sodium chicken or vegetable broth

1 medium onion, thinly sliced

1 medium diced red bell pepper 2 medium diced tomatoes

1 tablespoon fresh basil, chopped 2 tablespoons fresh parsley, chopped

Season with salt and pepper to taste.

Directions:

1. Slice the onion and set aside for 5 minutes to bring out its beneficial properties.

2. In a skillet, heat 2 tablespoons broth. When the broth starts to steam, add the onions and bell pepper.

3. Combine 12 cup broth, cod fillets, and tomatoes in a mixing bowl.

4. Cover and cook for 3-5 minutes over medium heat, or until the fish is done.

5. Season with salt and pepper to taste and add chopped basil and parsley.

Miso Salmon

The health-promoting omega-3 fatty acids, of which salmon is an excellent source, are among the fats that are important in Healthy Weight Loss. Enjoy this flavorful salmon recipe that takes little time to prepare.

Ingredients:

a third of a pound of salmon, cut into two pieces

1 tablespoon light miso

1 tablespoon Dijon mustard

3 tablespoons mirin* 1 tablespoon minced fresh ginger

1 teaspoon rice vinegar * Japanese rice cooking wine, available in the Asian section of the market

Directions:

1. Preheat the broiler with the rack in the center of the oven. Heat a stainless steel or cast iron skillet large enough to hold the salmon over high heat (about 10 minutes).

2. To make the glaze, combine miso, Dijon mustard, mirin, ginger, and vinegar. Coat the salmon generously with the mixture.

3. Remove the pan from the broiler and place the salmon in it.

Depending on the thickness of the salmon.

4. Boil 2 quarts of water while the salmon is cooking.
Boil for 3 minutes after adding the Swiss chard.

Quick Broiled Salmon with Ginger Mint Salsa

Variety is essential for Healthy Weight Loss. This delicious salsa goes especially well with salmon.

Ingredients:

¼ pound salmon fillet, cut in half

2 teaspoon lemon juice

Season with salt and pepper to taste.

To taste, extra virgin olive oil

Salsa

1 ripe tomato,

½ cup green onions, minced

1 teaspoon ginger, minced

2 teaspoons fresh mint, minced

1 teaspoon lime juice

Season with salt and pepper to taste.

Directions:

1. Preheat the broiler and heat an all-stainless-steel skillet (make sure the handle is also stainless steel) or cast iron pan for about 10 minutes to get it very hot. The pan should be 5 to 7 inches away from the heat.

2. Season the salmon with 2 teaspoons fresh lemon juice, salt, and pepper. (You can Quick Broil with the skin on; it just takes a minute or two longer.

After cooking, the skin will easily peel off.)

3. Remove pan from heat with a hot pad and place salmon on hot pan, skin side down. Return the pan to the broiler. Remember that it's cooking quickly on both sides, so it'll be done quickly, usually in 7 minutes depending on thickness. Check for doneness with a fork. When cooked, it will flake easily. Salmon tastes best when it is still pink on the inside.

4. Combine all salsa ingredients while the salmon is cooking.

5. When the salmon is done, spoon the salsa over it.

6. Top with mint and a drizzle of extra virgin olive oil.

Salmon with Dill Sauce

A traditional dish that adds flavor and nutrition to your Healthy Weight Loss Plan.

Salmon is a great source of those hard-to-find omega-3 fatty acids.

Enjoy!

Ingredients:

Salmon fillet, 1/3 pound, cut in half

1 teaspoon lemon juice

Season with salt and pepper to taste.

Dill Dressing

4 oz plain low-fat yogurt

1 medium seeded and diced cucumber

1 tablespoon chopped fresh dill weed

Season with salt and pepper to taste.

Directions:

1. Preheat the broiler to high and heat an all-stainless-steel skillet (make sure the handle is also stainless steel) or cast iron pan for about 10 minutes to get it very hot. The pan should be 5 to 7 inches away from the heat.

2. Season the salmon with 1 teaspoon lemon juice, salt, and pepper. (You can Quick Broil with the skin on; it just takes a minute or two longer. After cooking, the skin will easily peel off.)

3. Remove pan from heat with a hot pad and place salmon on hot pan, skin side down. Return the pan to the broiler. Remember that it's cooking quickly on both sides, so it'll be done quickly, usually in 7 minutes depending on thickness. Check for doneness with a fork. When cooked, it will flake easily. Salmon tastes best when it is still pink on the inside. After the salmon has finished cooking, drizzle it with the remaining 1 teaspoon lemon juice.

4. Drizzle dill sauce over the salmon.

Mustard with Salmon

Mustard adds a tangy flavor to omega-3-rich salmon, making it an excellent addition to your Healthy Weight Loss menu.

Ingredients:

¼ pound salmon fillet (cut in half)

2 teaspoon lemon juice

Season with salt and pepper to taste.

1 tablespoon Dijon mustard

Directions:

1. Preheat the broiler and heat an all-stainless-steel skillet (make sure the handle is also stainless steel) or cast iron pan for about 10 minutes to get it very hot. The pan should be 5 to 7 inches away from the heat.

2. Before broiling, rub salmon fillets with fresh lemon juice, salt, and pepper, and spread with Dijon mustard. (You can Quick Broil with the skin on; it just takes a minute or two longer. After cooking, the skin will easily peel off.)

3. Remove pan from heat with a hot pad and place salmon on hot pan, skin side down. Return the pan to the broiler. Keep in mind that it's cooking quickly on both sides, so it'll be done in about 5 minutes. Check for doneness with a fork. When cooked, it will flake easily.

Salmon tastes best when it is still pink on the inside. Cooking time is calculated at 10 minutes per inch of thickness.

Seared Asian Tuna

This nutrient-rich and flavorful Asian-inspired dish can be prepared in minutes and is high in B vitamins, selenium, and protein.

Ingredients:

4 ounces tuna, cut into two pieces

2 tablespoons mirin* 1 tablespoon fresh squeezed lemon juice

2 tablespoons tamari (soy sauce)

1 tablespoon minced fresh ginger

6 tablespoons minced scallions

* Japanese rice cooking wine, found in the Asian section of the market, to taste

Directions:

1. For 2 minutes, heat a 10-12 inch stainless steel skillet over medium-high heat.

2. While the pan is heating up, rub the tuna with 1 tablespoon lemon juice, season with salt and white pepper, and prepare the ginger and scallions.

3. Cook the tuna in a preheated skillet for 1-2 minutes on each side, depending on thickness, before removing from skillet. Seared tuna tastes best when it's medium rare.

4. Reduce the heat to medium and add the remaining ingredients to the pan in the order listed, cooking for 1 minute. Season with salt and pepper to taste.

Pour over tuna before serving.

Spicy Asian Shrimp

Shrimp is a good source of vitamin D, a vitamin that has recently gained popularity due to its importance in bone health. This recipe is not only low in calories, but it will get you a long way toward meeting your daily vitamin D requirements.

Ingredients:

3 oz. medium-sized peeled and deveined shrimp

2 tablespoons + 1 tablespoon fresh lemon juice

Season with salt and pepper to taste.

3 tbsp chicken or vegetable broth (low sodium)

2 chopped medium garlic cloves

1/8 teaspoon of red pepper flakes

¼ cup of orange juice

1 tablespoon minced fresh ginger

½ tablespoons extra virgin olive oil

Directions:

1. Chop garlic and set aside for 5 minutes to improve its health-promoting properties.

Peel and devein the shrimp.

3. Season the shrimp with 2 tablespoons lemon juice, salt, and pepper.

4. In a stainless steel skillet, heat 3 TBS broth over medium-low heat.

5. When the broth starts to steam, add the shrimp, red pepper flakes, orange juice, and ginger and sauté for a few minutes. Frequent stirring is required. After 2 minutes, flip the shrimp and add the garlic. Cook until the shrimp are pink and opaque all the way through (approximately 3 minutes). Shrimp cook quickly, so keep an eye on the cooking time. If overcooked, they become tough.

6. Toss with the remaining 1 tablespoon lemon juice and extra virgin olive oil.

Thai Scallops (or Shrimp) with Basil

This Thai-inspired Healthy Weight Loss dish is full of nutrients and flavor.

Ingredients:

¼ cup chicken or vegetable broth (low sodium)

2 cups green beans, 1 inch lengths

1 cup sliced fresh red bell peppers

1 teaspoon grated ginger

1 tsp garlic

¼ cup of coconut milk

1 tablespoon Thai curry paste

¼ pound medium raw shrimp or scallops

¼ cup chopped fresh basil

½ cup sunflower seeds

Directions:

1. Covered sauté green beans in 3 TBS broth for 3 minutes.

2. Add bell peppers and cook for 3 minutes more, covered.

3. Combine 1 teaspoon Thai curry paste, garlic, ginger, and coconut milk in a mixing bowl. Cook for 3-5 minutes.

4. Cook for another 3 minutes, uncovered, with the shrimp, basil, and sunflower seeds.

Dips and Side Vegetables Recipes

1 Minute Spinach

Enjoy this quick and easy addition to your Healthy Weight Loss Plan that is high in health-promoting nutrients like vitamin A, K, C, manganese, and folate.

Ingredients:

1 pound fresh spinach

1 teaspoon lemon juice

1 medium pressed or chopped fresh garlic

1 tablespoon of extra virgin olive oil

To taste, season with salt and cracked black pepper.

Optional: tomato, chopped

Directions:

1. Chop or press garlic and set aside for 5 minutes to extract its health-promoting properties.

2. In a large pot, bring lightly salted water to a rapid boil.

3. Remove the stems from the spinach leaves and thoroughly clean them. This is easily accomplished by leaving the spinach bundled and cutting off the stems all at once. Spinach leaves should be thoroughly rinsed because they often contain a lot of soil.

4. Cook spinach for 1 minute in boiling water.

5. Drain and press excess water out. While the spinach is still hot, combine the remaining ingredients.

3-Minute Guacamole

Guacamole is a popular condiment in Mexican and Southwestern cuisines. It only takes 3 minutes to incorporate this simple version into your Healthy Weight Loss Plan for an extra boost of vitamins A, C, and K.

Ingredients:

½ medium avocado

1 tablespoon lemon juice

12 cup cilantro leaves

Season with salt and pepper to taste.

Directions:

With a fork, mash the avocado and combine it with the remaining ingredients.

Swiss Chard

Swiss chard is one of the most nutrient-dense foods you can incorporate into your Healthy Weight Loss Eating Plan. It's a good source of vitamins A, C, K, magnesium, and manganese, and it goes well with almost any meal.

Ingredients:

1 pound chopped Swiss chard

1 medium garlic clove, chopped or pressed

1 tablespoon of extra virgin olive oil

1 teaspoon lemon juice

Season with salt and black pepper to taste.

Directions:

1. Chop or press garlic for 5 minutes to release its health-promoting properties.

2. Fill a large (3-quart) pot halfway with water. Before adding the Swiss chard, make sure the water is rapidly boiling.

3. Remove the tough bottom part of the Swiss chard stems.

4. Chop the leaves and place them in the boiling water. Do not conceal.

Cook for 3 minutes, starting when you place the Swiss chard in the boiling water.

5. Carefully remove the chard from the water, place it in a colander, and squeeze out any excess water.

6. Toss with lemon juice, olive oil, salt, and pepper in a serving dish.

5-Minute Broccoli

Broccoli, like other cruciferous vegetables, provides not only a good source of vitamins A, C, K, and folate, but also health-promoting sulphur compounds that help your liver detoxify potentially toxic substances.

Ingredients:

1 pound broccoli

½ tablespoons extra virgin olive oil

2 teaspoon lemon juice

2 garlic cloves

Season with salt and pepper to taste.

Directions:

1. Pour 2 inches of water into the bottom of the steamer.

2. While the steamer is heating up, cut the broccoli florets into quarters. Peel the stems and cut them into 14-inch pieces. Allow the florets and stems to sit for 5 minutes to release their hidden health benefits.

3. Chop or press garlic and set aside for 5 minutes.

4. If using stems, steam them for 2 minutes before adding the florets. 5 minutes of steaming florets

5. Place in a bowl. While the broccoli is still hot, toss it with the remaining ingredients.

5 Minutes Mustard Brussels Sprouts

Even if you've never liked Brussels sprouts, I think you'll enjoy adding this recipe to your Healthy Weight Loss menu. They, like their cousins broccoli and kale, are high in sulphur compounds, which are beneficial to the liver. And they only take a few minutes to make. Enjoy!

Ingredients:

1 pound Brussels sprouts

½ tablespoons extra virgin olive oil

1 teaspoon lemon juice

2 medium garlic cloves, chopped or pressed

1 tablespoon Dijon mustard

1 teaspoon honey

Season with salt and black pepper to taste.

Directions:

1. Pour 2 inches of water into the bottom of the steamer.

2. While the steamer is heating up, cut the Brussels sprouts into quarters and set aside for at least 5 minutes to bring out the hidden health benefits.

3. Chop or press garlic and set aside for at least 5 minutes to allow the health-promoting properties to emerge.

4. Cook for 5 minutes the Brussels sprouts.

5. Place in a bowl. Toss the Brussels sprouts with the remaining ingredients while they are still hot.

5 Minutes Cauliflower with Turmeric

Turmeric in this recipe adds not only flavor but also anti-inflammatory protection to your Healthy Weight Loss Plan.

Ingredients:

1 pound cauliflower

5 tbsp chicken or vegetable broth (low sodium)

1 teaspoon turmeric

½ tablespoons extra virgin olive oil

2 teaspoon lemon juice

2 medium garlic cloves, pressed or chopped

Season with salt and pepper to taste.

Directions:

1. Quarter the cauliflower florets and set aside for 5 minutes to bring out their hidden health benefits.

2. Set aside for 5 minutes after pressing or chopping the garlic.

3. In a stainless steel skillet over medium heat, heat 5 tablespoons broth.

4. When the broth starts to steam, add the cauliflower. Cover cauliflower with turmeric and set aside. Cook for no more than 5 minutes for al dente cauliflower.

5. Place in a bowl. Toss the cauliflower with the remaining ingredients while it is still hot for added flavor.

5-Minute Collard Greens

Collard greens are one of the best plant-based calcium sources, providing nearly as much as a cup of milk while containing half the calories and almost no fat! It's no surprise that they're an excellent addition to your Healthy Weight Loss Eating Plan.

Ingredients:

1 pound collard greens

1 tablespoon of extra virgin olive oil

1 teaspoon lemon juice

1 garlic clove, chopped

Season with salt and pepper to taste.

Directions:

1. Pour 2 inches of water into the bottom of the steamer.

2. Chop collard greens and set aside for 5 minutes to bring out their hidden health benefits while the steamer heats up.

3. Mince the garlic and set aside for at least 5 minutes.

4. Steam for 5 minutes the greens.

5. Place in a bowl. To add more flavor, toss the collard greens with the remaining ingredients while they are still hot.

5-Minute Italian Kale

With this delicious and simple recipe, you can incorporate kale into your Healthiest Way of Eating in a matter of minutes. Kale is one of the healthiest vegetables available, with one serving providing an excellent source of the antioxidant vitamins A and E.

Enjoy!

Ingredients:

1 pound (Lacinato) Italian kale (or any variety)

2 teaspoon lemon juice

1 medium garlic clove, pressed or chopped

12 tablespoons extra virgin olive oil

Season with salt and black pepper to taste.

Directions:

1. Chop garlic and set aside for 5 minutes to allow its health-promoting properties to develop.

2. Bring 2 inches of water to a boil in the bottom of the steamer.

3. While the water is heating up, cut the kale leaves into 12-inch slices and then crosswise. Slice the stems into 14-inch slices. Allow kale to sit for at least 5 minutes to bring out its beneficial properties.

4. When the water begins to boil, place the kale in the steamer basket and cover. 5 minutes of steaming.

5. Transfer to a mixing bowl and toss with remaining ingredients. Cook the kale while it is still hot for the best flavor.

5-Minute Mediterranean Medley

This is an excellent way to prepare a variety of vegetables and add more nutrition to your Healthy Weight Loss menu in the time it takes to prepare just one. Use this method to prepare a variety of your favorite vegetables.

Ingredients:

3 cups broccoli florets, quartered

3 cups chopped kale

1 medium carrot, sliced

2 garlic cloves, chopped or pressed

1 tablespoon of extra virgin olive oil

2 teaspoon lemon juice

Season with salt and pepper to taste.

Directions:

1. Pour 2 inches of water into the bottom of the steamer.

2. While the steam in the steamer is heating up, cut the broccoli and chop the kale and set aside for at least 5 minutes to bring out the hidden health benefits.

3. Chop or press garlic and set aside for at least 5 minutes to allow its health-promoting properties to emerge.

4. Cut carrots 14 inch thick.

5 minutes, steam broccoli, kale, and carrots.

6. Place in a bowl. Toss the vegetables with the remaining ingredients while they are still hot.

Garlic Dip

This recipe is ideal as an appetizer before dinner or as a snack at any time of day. Garlic not only has a delicious flavor, but it also adds extra antibacterial and antioxidant protection to your Healthy Weight Loss menu.

Ingredients:

2 cups garbanzo beans, cooked or canned

1 tablespoon lemon juice

¼ cup chicken or vegetable broth 3 chopped garlic cloves

2 tablespoons extra virgin olive oil

Season with salt and pepper to taste.

Directions:

In a blender, combine all of the ingredients and blend until smooth. Serve with your preferred crudités.

Healthy Mashed Sweet Potatoes

This full-flavored sweet potato dish is quick and easy to make, and it adds a healthy and unique twist to your Healthy Weight Loss Plan. In fact, one serving of this recipe has only 98 calories but contains 249% of your daily value (DV) of vitamin A. Enjoy!

Ingredients:

2 medium sweet potatoes or yams, peeled and thinly sliced for quick cooking

2 tablespoons fresh orange juice

1 tablespoon of extra virgin olive oil

Season with salt and white pepper to taste.

Directions:

1. In a steamer with a tight-fitting lid, bring lightly salted water to a boil.

2. Covered steam peeled and sliced sweet potatoes for about 10 minutes, or until tender.

3. Mash with a potato masher, then add the remaining ingredients.

Healthy Saut é ed Crimini Mushrooms

Enjoy this simple recipe that goes well with many of your favorite dishes and is an excellent addition to your Healthy Weight Loss Plan. Along with the great flavor of crimini mushrooms, you'll be getting a healthy dose of selenium, vitamin B12, and copper.

Ingredients:

1 pound sliced crimini mushrooms 3 tablespoons low-sodium chicken or vegetable broth

Season with salt and pepper to taste.

Directions:

1. In a stainless steel skillet, heat 3 tablespoons broth over medium heat.

2. Add the sliced mushrooms and sauté for 3 minutes once the broth begins to steam. As they cook, they will expel liquid. Because crimini mushrooms are less watery than other button mushrooms, stir constantly for the last 4 minutes. The liquid evaporates, and the mushrooms turn golden brown but are not burned.

3. Season with salt and pepper to taste.

Healthy Sauté ed Red Cabbage

Ingredients:

1 small head sliced red cabbage

5 tbsp low-sodium vegetable or chicken broth

1 tablespoon lemon juice

½ tablespoons extra virgin olive oil

1 garlic clove, chopped

Season with salt and pepper to taste.

Directions:

1. Chop garlic and set aside for 5 minutes to bring out its health benefits.

2. In a large skillet, heat 3 tablespoons broth. When the broth starts to steam, add the mushrooms and cook for 2 minutes, stirring constantly.

3. Cook for 5 minutes more after adding 5 tablespoons broth and the sliced cabbage.

4. Place in a bowl. Toss the vegetables with the remaining ingredients while they are still hot for added flavor.

Mediterranean Hummus

This Middle Eastern dish would make an excellent appetizer or snack on your Healthy Weight Loss menu. Its high protein and fiber content helps to satisfy your hunger and keep you feeling full between meals.

Ingredients:

2 cups garbanzo beans, cooked (or 15 oz can)

2 tablespoons low-sodium chicken broth

1 tablespoon + 2 tablespoons extra virgin olive oil

2 chopped garlic cloves

1 tablespoon tahini (sesame butter)

1 tablespoon lemon juice

Season with salt and pepper to taste.

Directions:

1. In a blender or food processor, combine garbanzo beans, chicken broth, 1 tablespoon extra virgin olive oil, garlic, tahini, and lemon juice. As the mixture is blending, drizzle in the 2 TBS olive oil a little at a time through the feed hole.

2. Season with salt and pepper to taste.

Serve each hummus serving with crudités.

Desserts Recipes

Fresh Berry Dessert with Yogurt and Chocolate

Because healthy weight loss is not about deprivation, a tasty dessert is a great way to treat yourself—and it's also nutritious!

Ingredients:

1 fresh 8-oz basket strawberries or raspberries

8 oz vanilla non-fat yogurt

2 oz dark chocolate, net weight

Directions:

1. Combine berries and yogurt in a mixing bowl.

2. Melt chocolate in a double boiler over medium heat. Drizzle melted chocolate over berries and yogurt in individual bowls.

3. For a more formal presentation, pour a pool of yogurt onto a plate and arrange berries on top. Drizzle the chocolate over the berries.

Ginger Pineapple

Fruit is an excellent way to satisfy your sweet tooth without adding a lot of calories to your Weight Loss Plan. The ginger adds a zing to this recipe, which has only 58 calories and is high in vitamin C and manganese.

Ingredients:

½ medium pineapple slices

1 teaspoon fresh ginger, finely minced

Directions:

1. Peel and cut the pineapple into 1-inch chunks.

2. Combine pineapple and minced ginger in a bowl and chill for half an hour.

Orange Treat

This simple dessert exemplifies how a dessert can be flavorful, nutritious, and low in calories. For only 82 calories, you get a tangy flavor as well as a good source of fiber and vitamins.

Ingredients:

½ teaspoon grated lemon rind* 12 teaspoon fresh lemon juice

2 tablespoons honey

2 tbsp. nonfat yogurt

2 large oranges

Optional: Garnish with orange zest

Directions:

1. In a small mixing bowl, combine the lemon rind, lemon juice, and honey.

2. Whisk in the yogurt thoroughly.

3. Peel and cut the orange into individual sections. Make certain that the membrane covering is removed from each section. Crosswise cut the sections into thirds. Divide the mixture between two dessert bowls.

4. Drizzle the sauce over the oranges.

*If possible, use organic lemon zest.